Ease the Mind:
45 Simple Strategies for Stress and Anxiety Relief

Practical Tools for a Calmer, Happier Life

By
Melanie J Nadler

Table of Contents

Introduction

Hello and welcome to my book on stress and anxiety awareness, management, and well-being. My name is Melanie J Nadler, and I am thrilled to have you here with me. As someone who has personally struggled with stress and anxiety, I understand the toll it can take on one's life. My goal with this book is to provide you with the necessary tools and techniques to effectively manage and overcome these challenges. Throughout our journey together, we will explore various methods to improve your overall well-being and find peace of mind. As your guide and support, I am dedicated to helping you achieve a happier and healthier life. Thank you for choosing to embark on this important path of self-care with me. Let's begin!

Stress and anxiety are common struggles in today's fast-paced world, and their negative impact on our well-being cannot be ignored. However, there are simple, holistic ways to manage and reduce stress in our daily lives. Incorporating deep breathing exercises, meditation, regular physical activity, and sufficient sleep can bring a sense of calm and freedom from stress. It's also important to connect with loved ones, set boundaries, and make time for hobbies and self-care. Remember, managing stress is a personal journey, and what works for one person may not work for another. By trying out a variety of techniques and finding what works best for us individually, we can achieve a sense of total freedom from stress and anxiety. So take the time to explore these 45 tips and techniques and find what brings you the most peace and balance in your life.

When it comes to making positive changes in our lives, it's crucial to start small and choose techniques that feel attainable and realistic for our individual situations. The tips and techniques I will be sharing are all designed to be bite-sized and easily integrated into your daily routine. It's important not to feel overwhelmed and attempt to implement all of them at once. Instead, take a gradual and intentional approach by selecting the ones that resonate with you and feel achievable. With this method, these techniques have the potential to create long-lasting and significant transformations in your life.

Stress and anxiety are two prevalent challenges that impact a large portion of the population. To gain a deeper understanding of these conditions, we will delve into their underlying causes and how they can manifest in our daily lives. By recognizing the signs and symptoms of stress and anxiety, we can take proactive steps towards managing and overcoming these overwhelming emotions. Furthermore, we will explore methods for cultivating inner resilience, which can aid in effectively coping with the various stressors and difficulties of life. Join us on this journey as we explore this crucial topic and acquire valuable tools for managing stress and anxiety.

Stress and anxiety are common experiences for many people and can manifest in both physical and psychological symptoms. Stress can be triggered by various demands on the brain and body, while anxiety is characterized by feelings of fear, worry, and unease. While stress and anxiety can be helpful in the short term, prolonged and excessive levels can negatively impact daily life. It is important to be aware of the symptoms, as they can vary from person to person, and may include stomach aches, muscle tension, headaches, rapid breathing, sweating, and changes in appetite and sleep patterns. If these symptoms begin to interfere with daily life, it may indicate a need for further support and attention.

It's important to recognize that stress and anxiety can have a significant impact on our mental and emotional well-being, in addition to physical symptoms. These can manifest as feelings of impending doom, panic, and nervousness, particularly in social settings. They can also make it difficult to concentrate and cause irrational anger and restlessness. While a little stress every now and then is normal, chronic stress can lead to serious health problems such as mental health disorders, cardiovascular disease, obesity, menstrual problems, sexual dysfunction, skin and hair issues, and gastrointestinal problems. It's essential to address and manage stress effectively to prevent these issues from occurring or worsening. Seeking support and implementing healthy coping mechanisms can help alleviate stress and improve overall health and well-being.

Stress and anxiety are common issues that can affect individuals in various ways. One of the main causes of stress and anxiety is work, with 40% of workers reporting that their job is a significant source of stress. This can be due to factors such as being unhappy in their job, heavy workloads, and poor management. Additionally, life stressors such as the death of a loved one, financial obligations, and traumatic events can also contribute to stress and anxiety. It's important to identify these triggers and find ways to cope with them in order to maintain a healthy well-being. By recognizing the causes of stress and anxiety, we can take steps to reduce their impact and improve our overall quality of life.

Stress can often stem from our own internal thoughts and worries rather than external factors. Our fears and uncertainties can create a constant state of stress and anxiety, and our attitudes and perceptions can greatly impact our stress levels. Additionally, having unrealistic expectations and facing change can also contribute to increased stress. It's important to recognize these factors and find healthy ways to cope with and manage our stress levels in order to maintain our overall well-being. By addressing these internal sources of stress, we can work towards creating a more peaceful and balanced mindset.

What is Stress Management?

The Gale Encyclopaedia of medicine 2008 states that stress management is:

(a) "set of techniques and programs intended to help people deal more effectively with stress in their lives by analysing the specific stressors and taking positive actions to minimize their effects."

In today's fast-paced world, stress has become a common occurrence for many individuals. While it's unrealistic to aim for a completely stress-free life, there are various ways to manage and reduce stress levels. Popular examples of stress management techniques include meditation, yoga, and exercise, and we will explore these in detail to ensure there is something that works for everyone. However, before delving into specific techniques, it's important to recognize that stress is a natural human response and not always negative. Nonetheless, identifying and managing stress can greatly benefit our overall well-being. In fact, The American Psychological Association offers 7 tips to support individuals in creating a stress management plan, and these will be discussed before diving into my own 45 stress management techniques.

1. Understand your stress
How do you stress? It can be different for everybody. By understanding what stress looks like for you, you can be better prepared, and reach for your stress management toolbox when needed.

2. Identify your stress sources
What causes you to be stressed? Be it work, family, change or any of the other potential thousand triggers.

3. Learn to recognize stress signals
We all process stress differently so it's important to be aware of your individual stress symptoms. What are your internal alarm bells? Low tolerance, headaches, stomach pains or a combination from the above 'Symptoms of stress'

4. Recognize your stress strategies

What is your go-to tactic for calming down? These can be behaviours learned over years and sometimes aren't the healthy option. For example, some people cope with stress by self-medicating with alcohol or overeating.

5. Implement healthy stress management strategies

It's good to be mindful of any current unhealthy coping behaviours so you can switch them out for a healthy option. For example, if overeating is your current go to, you could practice meditation instead, or make a decision to phone a friend to chat through your situation. The American Psychological Association suggest that switching out one behaviour at a time is most effective in creating positive change.

6. Make self-care a priority

When we make time for ourselves, we put our well-being before others. This can feel selfish to start, but it is like the aeroplane analogy—we must put our own oxygen mask on before we can assist others. The simplest things that promote well-being, such as enough sleep, food, downtime, and exercise are often the ones overlooked.

7. Ask for support when needed

If you're feeling overwhelmed, reach out to a friend or family member you can talk to. Speaking with a healthcare professional can also reduce stress and help us learn healthier coping strategies.

My 45 tips and techniques for reducing stress and anxiety effortlessly

Stress and anxiety are common struggles for many people, but thankfully, there are many techniques and tips that can help manage and alleviate these feelings. First and foremost, it's important to recognize the signs and symptoms of stress and anxiety, such as racing thoughts, increased heart rate, and muscle tension. Then, it's helpful to find healthy ways to cope, such as exercise, deep breathing, and mindfulness practices. In addition, setting boundaries, learning to say no, and prioritizing self-care can also greatly reduce stress and anxiety levels. It's also important to seek support from friends, family, or a professional therapist if needed. By incorporating these 45 stress and anxiety management tips and techniques into your daily routine, you can work towards a happier and more balanced life.

1. Yoga.

Yoga is a popular mind-body practice that has numerous benefits for both physical and mental health. By combining physical poses, controlled breathing, and meditation or relaxation, yoga has been shown to reduce stress, lower blood pressure, and lower heart rate. One of the great things about yoga is that it can be practiced by almost anyone, regardless of age, ability, or fitness level. This practice brings together physical and mental disciplines, helping to achieve a peaceful state of mind and body. It can be a valuable tool for managing stress and anxiety, which is why it has become so popular in today's fast-paced world. With many styles, forms, and intensities, there is a type of yoga for everyone. For those looking for a slower pace and easier movements, Hatha yoga is a great choice.

However, all styles of yoga can provide benefits and it ultimately comes down to personal preference.

The practice of hatha yoga, and most general yoga classes, includes three core components: poses, breathing, and meditation or relaxation. Poses, also known as asanas, involve a series of movements that aim to increase strength and flexibility. These movements can range from simple lying-down postures to challenging positions that push the physical limits. Breathing is another key element of yoga, with the belief that controlling one's breath can lead to better control over the body and a quieter mind. Lastly, yoga often incorporates meditation or relaxation techniques, helping individuals to become more mindful and present without judgment. These core components make up the foundation of a yoga practice, promoting physical and mental well-being.

Yoga has gained immense popularity over the years, and for good reason. Not only is it a great form of physical exercise, but it also has potential health benefits that can greatly improve one's overall well-being. Numerous studies have shown that regular yoga practice can reduce stress and anxiety, while enhancing mood and promoting relaxation. Additionally, it can improve balance, flexibility, range of motion, and strength, making it an effective form of fitness. Furthermore, yoga has been linked to managing chronic conditions, such as heart disease, high blood pressure, depression, pain, anxiety, and insomnia. So why not give yoga a try and experience its potential health benefits for yourself?

Before starting any yoga practice, it's important to consult with a trained instructor and your healthcare provider to ensure safety and avoid potential risks. While yoga is generally considered safe for most healthy individuals, there are certain conditions or situations that may increase the risk. These include a herniated disk, a history of blood clots, eye conditions like glaucoma, pregnancy (although it can be practiced with caution), severe balance problems, severe osteoporosis, and uncontrolled blood pressure. In these cases, modifications and precautions may need to be taken, such as avoiding certain poses or stretches. It's also important to listen to your body and consult with your doctor if you experience any symptoms or concerns during your practice. With the right guidance and precautions, yoga can provide numerous benefits and help improve overall health and well-being.

As a yoga practitioner, it's important to listen to your body and honour its limits. Whether you prefer hot yoga or gentle flow, there is no need to force yourself into every pose. If a particular pose feels uncomfortable or if you are unable to hold it for the full duration, it is perfectly acceptable to modify or skip it. A good yoga instructor will encourage you to explore your boundaries while also respecting them. Remember, yoga is a personal journey and it's important to honour your own body's needs and abilities.

2. Tai Chi

Originating in China, tai chi is a traditional form of exercise rooted in martial arts that involves slow, deliberate movements and controlled breathing techniques. Its physical and emotional benefits are well-documented, including a reduction in anxiety and depression, improved cognitive function, and potential management of symptoms related to chronic illnesses like fibromyalgia and COPD. Incorporating tai chi into your fitness routine can provide numerous health benefits for both the mind and body. So why not give it a try and experience the transformative effects of this ancient practice for yourself?

Tai chi, a mind-body exercise rooted in ancient Chinese martial arts, has been shown to have significant benefits for reducing stress and anxiety. In fact, a 2018 study compared the effects of tai chi to traditional exercises on stress-related anxiety and found that both forms of exercise provided similar benefits. However, tai chi stood out because it also incorporates elements of meditation and focused breathing, making it potentially superior to other forms of exercise for managing stress and anxiety. By combining physical movement with mental and emotional practices, tai chi offers a holistic approach to managing stress and promoting overall well-being.

Preliminary research has shown that regularly practicing Tai Chi can have a positive impact on individuals who struggle with anxiety and depression. This ancient form of martial arts involves slow, mindful movements and deep breathing, which is believed to have a calming effect on the nervous system and regulate mood hormones. By incorporating Tai Chi into your routine, you may experience an improvement in your overall mood and a reduction in symptoms associated with anxiety and depression. It's important to note that further research is needed, but the potential benefits of this practice make it worth considering for those struggling with mental health concerns.

Incorporating tai chi into your routine may have a positive impact on your sleep quality. A study focusing on young adults with anxiety prescribed two tai chi classes per week for 10 weeks found that participants experienced significant improvements in sleep quality compared to the control group. Not only did the tai chi group report better sleep, but they also saw a decrease in their symptoms. The benefits of tai chi extend to older adults as well, with one study showing that 2 months of twice-weekly tai chi classes resulted in improved sleep for older adults with cognitive impairment. By regularly practicing tai chi, individuals of all ages may experience more restful sleep and a decrease in related symptoms.

3. Qi gong.

Qi gong, a traditional Chinese practice, has been shown to have powerful effects on overall health and well-being. This system works by harmonizing and strengthening the functioning of internal organs and bodily systems. By increasing the flow of energy throughout the body, qi gong can have rejuvenating effects and is even believed to increase longevity. Beyond the physical benefits, qi gong also has a positive impact on mental and emotional states, inducing feelings of calm and balance. Overall, this holistic practice has a multi-faceted approach to improving one's health and can be a valuable addition to any wellness routine.

Qi gong is a gentle and effective movement practice that has been found to release tension in the body and increase the flow of blood and energy. This can have a nourishing effect on all parts of the body, helping to improve overall health and well-being. In addition, many students have reported feeling deeply relaxed and energized after a session of Qi gong, with some even experiencing a deeper and more restful sleep that night. By focusing on gentle movements and stretches, Qi gong allows individuals to release tension that may have built up over many years, resulting in a feeling of greater physical and mental ease.

In traditional Chinese medicine, it is believed that the energy flowing through our internal organs can be accessed and improved through specific movements of the extremities - our hands and feet. This is why stretching exercises, such as yoga and tai chi, have been used for centuries to promote the health and balance of the body's internal organs. By stretching and strengthening the arms and legs, we can improve the flow of energy and support the overall health of our organs. This ancient practice continues to be recognized and utilized in modern medicine as a holistic approach to maintaining optimal health.

In the practice of qi gong, the breath is of utmost importance. It should be relaxed, slow, and deep, originating from the diaphragm. This specific type of breathing has a powerful impact on the mind, promoting a sense of calmness and balance. This is especially beneficial in counteracting the negative effects of worry and stress. Even just a few minutes of qi gong can work wonders in alleviating stress whenever it arises. So the next time you start feeling overwhelmed, take a few moments to focus on your breath and practice qi gong to restore a sense of peace and harmony within your mind and body.

Qi gong, an ancient Chinese practice, offers a variety of benefits in its early stages of practice. As you become more attuned to your body, you will start to notice the more subtle and refined effects of qi gong. This includes improved balance, increased energy and focus, and a stronger mind-body connection. With consistent practice, you may also experience reduced stress and anxiety, improved circulation and immune function, and a deeper sense of inner peace. As you progress in your practice, these benefits will continue to grow and expand, helping you to live a more balanced and harmonious life. Give qi gong a try and discover the transformative power it can have on your mind, body, and spirit.

4. Meditation

Meditation is a widely recognized practice for relieving stress, utilized by individuals from all backgrounds. This ancient method can take various forms and may be incorporated with other spiritual practices, serving a variety of important purposes. One way meditation can be beneficial is as a quick and effective stress-relieving tool, helping to reverse the body's stress response and induce physical relaxation. Additionally, making meditation a part of your daily routine can aid in building resilience to stress. Lastly, in moments of emotional stress, meditation can be a helpful technique to regain centre and balance. By incorporating meditation into your life, you can experience its numerous benefits for managing stress and improving overall well-being.

Meditation has proven to be a powerful tool in reducing both physical and emotional stress. By bringing attention to your body and mind, you can release tension and anxiety, leaving you feeling rejuvenated and ready to tackle your day with a positive outlook. With consistent practice over time, the benefits of meditation can become even more profound. By triggering the body's relaxation response, meditation works to reverse the harmful effects of stress on the body. It allows the body to enter a state of calmness, promoting healing and preventing further damage caused by stress. Additionally, the quieting of stress-induced thoughts during meditation leads to a deep sense of relaxation in both the mind and body. This double dose of relaxation makes meditation a powerful tool for managing and reducing stress.

One of the many benefits of meditation is its ability to cultivate long-term resilience. Studies have shown that individuals who regularly practice meditation develop a heightened response to stress, allowing them to recover from difficult situations more easily and experience less overall stress in their daily lives. This can be attributed in part to the increase in positive mood that often accompanies meditation. Research has also shown that those who experience positive moods more frequently tend to be more resilient towards stress. Additionally, the brains of regular meditation practitioners have been found to undergo changes that lead to decreased reactivity towards stress. These findings highlight the significant impact that regular meditation practice can have on building resilience and managing stress in the long-term.

Incorporating meditation into your daily routine can have multiple benefits, including helping you to redirect your thoughts and combat negative thinking patterns, which can ultimately relieve stress. This practice allows you to take control of your stress response and reverse it, protecting you from the harmful effects of chronic stress. By simply dedicating a few minutes each day to meditation, you can experience a multitude of solutions for improving your overall well-being.

When practising meditation:
1. Your heart rate and breathing slow down
2. Your blood pressure normalises
3. You use oxygen more efficiently
4. Your immune function improves
5. You sweat less
6. Your adrenal glands produce less cortisol
7. Your mind ages at a slower rate
8. Your mind clears and your creativity increases

Meditation has been proven to have a powerful impact on our daily lives. Through regular practice, people are able to break free from harmful habits such as smoking, drinking, and drug use. In addition, meditation helps individuals combat rumination, allowing them to focus on the present and avoid letting negative thoughts ruin their day. This practice also helps people tap into their inner strength and build resilience, making it a valuable tool for a diverse range of individuals. Countless studies have shown the benefits of meditation, including reducing stress and promoting overall well-being. Incorporating meditation into your daily routine can have a positive and lasting impact on your life.

5. Take a break

Taking a break from the demands of everyday life, whether it be through holidays or short breaks, can bring many rewards. One of the most significant benefits is the reduction of stress that comes with being in a less demanding environment. Holidays provide us with a much-needed break from chronic stress, allowing us to physically and mentally restore ourselves to a healthier state. By breaking the cycle of stress, we can experience sharper thinking, increased creativity, and improved memory, all of which can positively impact our performance in all areas of life. This leads to a more fulfilling and enjoyable life, not just during the break, but also for a prolonged period after we return. Ultimately, taking time to rest and recharge is essential for our overall well-being and success.

While it may be easy to recognize when a holiday is needed, sometimes the stress we experience can sneak up on us, making it difficult to identify when we are at risk for overwhelm or burnout. We all respond to stress differently, so it's important to be aware of the signs of overwhelm that are unique to us. However, there are some common warning signs that can apply to most people. If you're experiencing any of the following, it may be a good idea to start planning some downtime, even if it's just a weekend staycation to recharge and relax feeling constantly tired and fatigued, difficulty concentrating, increased irritability or mood swings, frequent headaches or muscle tension, and a decrease in motivation or enjoyment of activities. Remember, taking breaks and allowing yourself time to recharge is essential for maintaining good mental and emotional well-being.

Signs that you should take a break:
1. Lack of energy
2. Lack of motivation
3. More frequent frustration
4. Feeling fuzzy headed
5. Mild health issues
6. Sleep disturbances due to stress

Taking care of our mental health is just as important as taking care of our physical health. It's crucial to listen to our bodies and recognize when we need a break in order to maintain our overall well-being. Whether it's a long vacation or a few minutes of self-care throughout the day, taking time to recharge and manage stress can help us function at our best. By disrupting the body's stress response cycle, we can avoid feeling overwhelmed and stay energized, motivated, and engaged in our work and relationships. So, if you're feeling burnt out, consider taking a holiday or mental health day to give yourself the break you need. After all, self-care is an essential part of maintaining a healthy and fulfilling life.

In our fast-paced world, it's important to take a break and prioritize self-care. While it may seem counterintuitive, taking time for yourself can actually help increase productivity and overall well-being. Some quick and easy options to incorporate self-care into your routine include going for a walk or bike ride, watching a movie, or even taking a 5–10-minute meditation break. By giving yourself a mental and physical break, you can recharge and come back to your tasks with renewed focus and energy. So don't forget to take some time for yourself – it's essential for a balanced and healthy life.

6. Positive thinking and stopping negative self-talk

How we view the world around us can have a profound impact on our lives, from our attitudes towards ourselves to our overall health and well-being. This is reflected in the age-old question: is your glass half empty or half full? Your answer to this question may indicate whether you have a more optimistic or pessimistic outlook on life. Research suggests that our personality traits, such as optimism and pessimism, can have a significant influence on our health. Studies have shown that positive thinking, which is often associated with optimism, is an important factor in managing stress effectively. Effective stress management, in turn, has been linked to numerous health benefits. For those who tend to have a more pessimistic mindset, there is hope. Positive thinking is a skill that can be learned, and it does not mean ignoring life's challenges. Rather, it means approaching them with a more positive and productive mindset, focusing on the best possible outcome rather than the worst. So, the next time someone asks if your glass is half empty or half full, remember that you have the power to choose a positive perspective and reap the benefits in your life.

In order to cultivate a positive outlook on life, it's important to pay attention to our self-talk. Self-talk refers to the continuous stream of thoughts that run through our minds, both consciously and unconsciously. These thoughts can either be positive or negative and can greatly influence our overall perspective. While some of our self-talk is based on logic and reason, other thoughts may stem from misconceptions or lack of information. Therefore, it's important to actively monitor and challenge our self-talk in order to promote a more positive mindset. By cultivating positive self-talk, we can become more optimistic and approach life with a more positive attitude.

Researchers continue to explore the effects of positive thinking and optimism on health. Health Benefits that positive thinking provide include:

1. Increased lifespan
2. Lower rates of depression
3. Lower rates of distress
4. Great resistance to the common cold
5. Better psychological and physical well-being
6. Better Cardiovascular health and reduced risk of death from cardiovascular disease.
7. Better coping skills during hardships and times of stress.

There are many health benefits associated with positive thinking, although it is still unclear exactly why this is the case. One theory suggests that having a positive outlook allows individuals to better cope with stressful situations, reducing the negative effects of stress on the body. The good news is, with practice, it is possible to transform negative thinking into positive thinking. This process may seem simple, but it does take time and effort to create a new habit. The first step is to identify areas in your life where you tend to have negative thoughts, whether it be work, your daily commute, or a relationship. From there, you can start small and focus on approaching one area with a more positive mindset. With determination and practice, you can become more optimistic and engage in positive thinking, leading to a healthier and happier life.

Taking a moment to evaluate our thoughts throughout the day is a great way to combat negative thinking. If we find ourselves stuck in a negative mindset, it's important to try and find a positive spin on our thoughts. Additionally, giving we permission to smile and laugh, even during difficult times, can help to reduce stress. Seeking humour in everyday situations can also bring a sense of levity and ease to our minds. Surrounding ourselves with positive and supportive individuals is crucial for managing stress in a healthy way. Negative people can often increase our stress levels and make us doubt our abilities, so it's important to seek out individuals who can provide helpful advice and feedback. By incorporating these practices into our daily lives, we can better manage stress and promote a more positive mindset.

One of the most important things to remember when it comes to self-talk is to treat yourself with the same kindness and encouragement that you would offer to anyone else. It's easy to be critical of ourselves, but this can have a negative impact on our self-esteem and overall well-being. Instead, when a negative thought arises, try to evaluate it rationally and respond with affirmations of your positive qualities. It can also be helpful to focus on things you are grateful for in your life. Changing negative self-talk habits takes time and effort, so don't expect to become an optimist overnight. However, with practice and persistence, your self-talk will become more positive and accepting, leading to a more optimistic outlook on life. This can also help you better handle everyday stress in a constructive way, contributing to the well-known benefits of positive thinking.

7. Hypnotherapy and self-hypnosis

Hypnosis may seem mysterious, but it is a powerful therapeutic tool that can help individuals overcome fears, manage pain, and reduce stress in their lives. It is important to remember to treat yourself with kindness and encouragement, and to respond to negative thoughts with positive affirmations. Practicing gratitude and focusing on the good in your life can also be beneficial for your overall well-being. While some may think of hypnosis as a way to control others, it is actually a collaborative process between a trained professional and a willing participant. Additionally, with self-hypnosis techniques, you can save time and money by learning to hypnotize yourself with your own voice or thoughts. Overall, hypnosis is a valuable tool that can be used for personal growth and self-improvement.

Hypnosis is a powerful tool for managing stress in multiple ways. Firstly, it can induce a deeply relaxed state that triggers the body's natural relaxation response, effectively reducing tension and preventing chronic stress-related health issues. Secondly, hypnosis can be used to implement healthy lifestyle changes that reduce overall stress levels, such as sticking to an exercise routine, maintaining a clutter-free home, and setting boundaries with others. Additionally, hypnosis can be used to alleviate anxiety in situations that typically cause stress, such as intimidating social interactions. Moreover, hypnosis can be an effective method for breaking negative habits that are used to cope with stress, such as smoking or overeating. By utilizing hypnosis for stress management, individuals can experience improved overall well-being and reduced stress levels.

The process of hypnosis is a powerful tool that can be utilized in a variety of ways. It involves entering a trance, or a state of deep relaxation and focus, similar to daydreaming or meditation. This state allows for suggestions to be made to the subconscious mind, resulting in effective results for the individual. One can seek out a trained professional for hypnotherapy, where they will guide and talk the person through the process. Alternatively, one can learn about hypnosis through books, videos, or articles and achieve results at home. This method is not only easy and cost-effective, but the results are long-lasting. Furthermore, there are minimal potential negative side effects, and it can provide multiple benefits simultaneously. In rare cases, upsetting information may arise from the subconscious mind, but this can be discussed and processed in therapy. Overall, hypnosis is a valuable tool that can be utilized for a variety of purposes and has the potential to bring about positive and lasting changes in one's life.

Hypnosis may not be suitable for everyone, as some individuals may have preconceived notions about the practice or struggle to enter the necessary trance-like state for suggestions to take effect. Additionally, some may find it challenging to make time for or fully focus on hypnosis as a stress management technique. In these cases, it may be beneficial to explore alternative methods for managing stress. It's important to find what works best for each individual, as everyone's needs and preferences are unique.

8. Visualisation and guided imagery techniques

Incorporating visualisation and imagery techniques into our daily routines can provide a powerful tool for reducing stress. By creating a vivid mental image of a serene and tranquil environment, we can help our minds and bodies to relax and let go of tension. These techniques are often paired with physical relaxation methods, such as progressive muscle relaxation or massage, in order to strengthen the connection between the visual image and the sensation of relaxation. The ultimate goal is to be able to easily conjure up feelings of calm and peace by simply visualising the serene setting, even without the use of physical relaxation techniques. By regularly practising guided imagery, we can train our minds to quickly access a state of relaxation whenever needed.

Guided imagery techniques are a valuable tool for relaxation due to their ability to distract the mind and redirect attention away from sources of stress. By focusing on an alternative and more peaceful environment, individuals are able to distance themselves from their stressors and enter a state of relaxation. These techniques provide non-verbal instructions to the body and unconscious mind, encouraging them to imagine and experience a sense of safety, peace, and beauty. This serves as a powerful suggestion to the mind and body, helping them to relax and release tension. Overall, guided imagery techniques are a highly effective way to induce relaxation and manage stress.

The use of imagery techniques can be likened to a form of guided meditation, where the ultimate goal is to teach individuals how to detach from their constantly shifting thoughts and instead cultivate a relaxed detachment that allows them to simply observe their thoughts and sensations. This meditative learning can be achieved through the repetitive practice of imagery techniques, allowing individuals to become more aware of their thoughts and learn to let them pass without becoming entangled in them. Through this process, individuals can gain a sense of calm and clarity, ultimately leading to a more peaceful and mindful state of being.

Guided imagery is a highly accessible technique, as it relies solely on one's imagination and ability to concentrate - skills that are always readily available (as long as one is not completely exhausted). However, as with any technique that requires mental focus, it is most effective when practiced without interruption. This allows for a deeper level of concentration and immersion in the guided imagery experience. By setting aside a specific time and place for guided imagery, individuals can create an environment that is conducive to relaxation and mental clarity. Whether it's a quiet corner of the house or a peaceful outdoor space, finding a distraction-free zone can greatly enhance the benefits of guided imagery. So next time you practice, make sure to eliminate any potential interruptions and create a serene setting for optimal results.

There is no single correct way to use visual imagery for stress relief. However, something similar to the following steps is often recommended:

Find a private space and make yourself comfortable.
Take a few slow deep breaths to centre your attention and calm yourself.
Close your eyes (if you haven't already)
imagine yourself in a beautiful location, where everything is as you would ideally have it. Some people visualise a beach, a mountain, a forest, or being in a favourite room sitting in a favourite chair.
Imagine yourself becoming calm and relaxed. Alternatively, imagine yourself smiling, feeling happy and having a good time.
Focus on the different sensory attributes present in your scene so as to make it more vivid in your mind. For instance, if you are imagining the beach, spend some time vividly imagining the warmth of the sun on your skin, the smell of the ocean, seaweed and salt spray; and the sound of the waves, wind and seagulls. The more you can invoke your senses, the more vivid the entire image will become. Remain with your scene, touring its various sensory aspects for five to 10 minutes or until you feel relaxed.

While relaxed, assure yourself that you can return to this place whenever you want to or need to relax.
Open your eyes again and then re-join your world.

9. Cognitive Reframing

In the face of potential stresses, our mindset can greatly impact our level of stress. That's where cognitive reframing comes in, a well-established technique recommended by psychologists. By consciously shifting our perspective and looking at things in a more positive light, we can minimize our stress and promote a sense of peace and control. This simple yet powerful tool can be used in various situations to help us better manage our emotions and navigate through challenges. With practice, cognitive reframing can become a natural and effective way to cope with stress and maintain a sense of balance in our lives.

Reframing is a powerful tool that can help us change our perspective and ultimately, our experience of a situation. By shifting the way we view something, we can turn a potentially stressful event into a challenge to be overcome with bravery or see a really bad day as a small bump in an otherwise wonderful life. We can also view negative events as opportunities for growth and learning. Reframing allows us to see the positive aspects of a situation and approach it with a more productive mindset. It is a valuable skill to have in both personal and professional settings, as it can help us navigate difficult situations with a more positive outlook. So the next time you're faced with a challenging event, try reframing it and see how it can change your experience.

In our fast-paced and demanding lives, stress can feel like a constant companion. However, there is a way to alter our perceptions of stress through re framing, which can help alleviate its negative effects and create a more positive life without making any major changes to our circumstances. By using re framing techniques, we can change our physical responses to stress because our body's stress response is often triggered by perceived stress rather than actual events. This means that by changing our perceptions, we can minimize the stresses we feel in our lives and ease the process of relaxation. From small annoyances to more serious situations, our stress response can remain triggered long after the initial event has passed, making it crucial to practice re framing and relaxation techniques in order to maintain a more positive and peaceful mindset.

10. Positive affirmations

In the journey towards personal growth and development, positive affirmations can be a powerful tool. By consciously choosing and repeating positive statements, we can reprogram our unconscious minds from negative thinking to a more positive outlook. These affirmations become a part of our thought patterns and perception of the world, working in a similar way to negative self-talk, but with a more beneficial impact. By incorporating positive affirmations into our daily routines, we can cultivate a more optimistic mindset and ultimately improve our overall well-being. So the next time you catch yourself engaging in negative self-talk, try replacing it with a positive affirmation and see the difference it can make in your life.

Positive self-talk can be a powerful tool in reducing stress, changing negative thinking patterns, and maintaining motivation. By creating a collection of personal statements, you can have a go-to resource for when you need a boost of confidence or a reminder of your strengths. It's important to use a conversational tone when writing these statements, as if you were talking to a close friend. Remember to avoid jargon and use everyday language that feels natural to you. Additionally, make sure to include specific examples and personal experiences to make your self-talk more relatable and effective. With these guidelines, you can create a powerful and personalized tool to support your mental well-being.

Before making any changes in your life, it's important to examine your intentions. What is the end goal you are trying to achieve? What behaviours, attitudes, and traits do you want to develop in order to reach that goal? Take the time to sit down and reflect on what truly matters to you. Consider journaling or brainstorming to get to the heart of what you want to create in your life. Whether it's finding more peace, adopting healthy habits, or becoming a better friend, knowing your intentions will help guide your actions and bring you closer to the life you desire.

When setting goals and manifesting our desires, it's important to use positive and present-tense statements. Instead of saying I want to feel more peaceful, phrase it as I am feeling more peaceful each day.

This subtle change can make a big difference in the way our subconscious mind receives and interprets the statement. By speaking as if our desires are already true, we are programming our mind to believe it and manifest it into reality. It's not about wanting something; it's about making it a reality. So take some time to craft positive and present-tense statements that reflect your goals and desires. This will help align your thoughts and actions with your intentions, ultimately leading to their manifestation.

When practicing positive affirmations, it's important to focus on what you want to see and experience, rather than what you want to avoid. Our minds may not register the negative aspect of a statement, so it's crucial to use positive language. For example, instead of saying I don't want to feel stress, or I've stopped feeling stressed, try saying I'm feeling peaceful. This way, your mind is solely focused on the desired outcome and not the unwanted feeling. By being intentional with your positive affirmations, you can effectively shift your mindset and manifest the positive experiences you desire.

When using positive affirmations, it's important to strike a balance between stretching your perspective and staying realistic. Your subconscious mind can benefit from affirmations that push you to grow and expand, but if they are too far-fetched, your inner judge will step in and discredit them. That's why it's crucial to choose affirmations that are hopeful and optimistic, but still believable to your subconscious mind. For example, affirmations like I am getting better and stronger every day may feel like too much of a stretch, while statements like I am learning from my mistakes or I am grateful for all that I have in my life may feel more attainable. It's important to experiment and find affirmations that resonate with you and feel genuine to your subconscious mind. With the right balance, positive affirmations can truly work wonders for your mindset and well-being.

Finding ways to reduce stress and increase peace and self-efficacy can be a challenging task. One way to get started is by seeking inspiration from others. Take a look at affirmations written by others that focus on promoting peaceful thoughts, feelings of safety, and a stronger sense of self-efficacy. Simple phrases such as I'm going to enjoy today, and I can handle whatever comes my way can serve as a great starting point for your own affirmations. Remember, finding what works best for you may take some time, so be patient and open to trying different techniques. With the help of others' affirmations and your own exploration, you can find ways to reduce stress and cultivate a more peaceful mindset.

Positive affirmations can be a powerful tool for self-improvement and personal growth. While it may feel awkward or silly at first, repeating positive statements to yourself can have a profound effect on your mindset and outlook. One fun way to incorporate affirmations into your daily routine is to create a collection of statements that resonate with you and display them in places where you'll see them often, such as your bathroom mirror or phone lock screen. You can also use affirmation cards or create a daily mantra to repeat to yourself. Another great idea is to involve a friend or family member and take turns sharing affirmations with each other. Whatever method you choose, introducing positive affirmations into your life can have a lasting impact on your mental and emotional well-being. So why not give it a try and see the positive changes it can bring to your life?

Repetition is a powerful tool when it comes to harnessing the power of affirmations. By regularly repeating affirmations to yourself, you can reinforce positive thoughts and beliefs in your mind. Whether it's mentally repeating them in the morning or evening, or saying them out loud, repetition can have a profound impact on your mindset. Saying affirmations out loud is especially effective as you are able to hear them more clearly and feel their impact on a deeper level. Make a habit of repeating your affirmations daily to see positive changes in your thoughts and attitudes.

Recording yourself reciting positive affirmations can be a powerful tool in improving your self-esteem and overall mindset. By using a calm tone and incorporating soothing background music, you can create a personalized recording that can be played during daily activities such as driving or getting ready in the morning. This do-it-yourself approach allows you to tailor the recording to your specific needs and can serve as a constant reminder of your worth and capabilities. With a self-made recording, you can take control of your self-talk and cultivate a more positive and empowering inner dialogue. So why not give it a try and see how this simple yet effective technique can make a difference in your life?

One simple and effective way to incorporate affirmations into your daily routine is by using post-its. These small sticky notes can be placed around your house in places where you are likely to see them, such as the fridge, bathroom mirror, or your desk. By placing affirmations on these post-its, you are giving yourself positive messages throughout the day. This technique can be used on its own or in combination with other affirmation techniques as a way to reinforce and strengthen your positive mindset. The visual reminder of the post-its can be a powerful tool in keeping you focused on your affirmations and boosting your confidence and self-belief. Give it a try and see how these small but mighty post-its can make a big impact on your daily mindset.

Self-hypnosis is a powerful tool for reinforcing affirmations and bringing about positive changes in your life. By utilizing self-hypnosis techniques, you can more effectively imprint your affirmations into your subconscious mind, resulting in faster and more lasting results. This process allows you to bypass the critical mind and access the subconscious, where true change can occur. By combining affirmations with self-hypnosis, you can supercharge your efforts towards achieving your goals and manifesting your desires. With regular practice, you can harness the power of self-hypnosis to create the life you truly want.

11. Social support

Research has shown that having close friends and family can have a significant impact on your overall health. Not only do these relationships provide emotional support during tough times, but they also help combat feelings of isolation and loneliness. That's why it's important to cultivate a strong social support network, made up of friends, family, and peers. While support groups can also be helpful in times of stress, a social support network is something that can be developed before any crisis occurs. It offers the reassurance of knowing that you have a support system in place whenever you need it. So don't wait until you're facing a difficult situation to focus on building and maintaining strong relationships with your loved ones. Start now and reap the many benefits of a strong social support network.

Maintaining a strong support network is crucial for our overall well-being. While it may seem tempting to isolate ourselves and handle our problems alone, studies have shown the negative effects of social isolation and loneliness on both our mental and physical health. Building relationships through simple actions like grabbing a coffee with a co-worker, chatting with a neighbour, or volunteering can greatly improve our ability to cope with stress, alleviate emotional distress, boost self-esteem, and promote good mental health. Furthermore, having a network of social support has been linked to lowering cardiovascular risks, promoting healthy behaviours, and encouraging adherence to treatment plans. So let's not underestimate the power of a simple conversation or visit, as they can have a significant impact on our overall health and well-being.

Building a strong social network can have a positive impact on your mental health and ability to cope with stress. One way to expand your social circle is by volunteering for a cause that aligns with your interests and values. This not only allows you to give back to your community, but also provides opportunities to meet like-minded individuals. Joining a gym or fitness group is another great way to make friends while prioritizing physical health. Additionally, taking a class through a local college or community education program can introduce you to others who share similar hobbies and interests.

Don't forget the power of social media in connecting with friends and family and consider exploring online communities specifically geared towards individuals going through challenging life changes. Just be sure to exercise caution and stick to reputable sites when arranging in-person meetings. With a little effort, you can build a strong support system to help you navigate life's ups and downs.

Maintaining strong relationships is a crucial aspect of a fulfilling life, and it takes effort and active involvement on both sides. Staying in touch with friends and family by answering phone calls, returning emails, and reciprocating invitations shows that you care about them and value your relationship. It's important to resist the urge to compete and instead be genuinely happy for your loved ones' successes. Being a good listener is also key in nurturing relationships; taking the time to listen and understand what is important to your friends and family shows that you value their thoughts and feelings. However, it's also important not to overdo it and overwhelm your loved ones with constant communication. Save those moments for when you truly need support. Remember to show your appreciation for your friends and family, and don't be afraid to give back and offer support when they need it. By following these suggestions, you can help strengthen and maintain the relationships that mean the most to you.

In order to build a strong social support network, it's important to keep in mind that the ultimate goal is to reduce your stress levels, not add to them. Pay attention to situations that seem to drain your energy and avoid spending too much time with individuals who are constantly negative and critical. Additionally, it's wise to steer clear of people who engage in unhealthy behaviours, such as alcohol or substance abuse. Taking the time to cultivate meaningful relationships and connections is a valuable investment in both your mental and physical well-being. So start reaching out to make new friends or strengthen the ones you already have. Whether you're the one receiving support or giving it, the rewards will be worth it in the long run.

12. Pets

While pet owners are familiar with the immediate joys of having a furry companion, the physical and mental health benefits of the human-animal bond are often overlooked. Only in recent years have studies delved into the scientific evidence of these benefits, shedding light on the positive impact that pets can have on our well-being. Whether it's the comfort and love that pets provide, the increased physical activity from walks and playtime, or the decrease in stress and anxiety, there's no denying that our animal companions bring numerous benefits to our lives. It's important to recognize and appreciate these benefits as we continue to enjoy the joys of pet ownership.

As humans, we have formed a strong bond with our pets, especially dogs. Over time, our pets have evolved to become incredibly in tune with our emotions and behaviours. While dogs can understand many of the words we use, they excel at interpreting our tone of voice, body language, and gestures. Like a loyal friend, they will look into our eyes to gauge our emotional state and try to understand our thoughts and feelings. This level of understanding and connection is what makes pets such important and valued companions in our lives. They are able to offer comfort, support, and companionship in a way that only a truly understanding and empathetic creature can.

It's no secret that owning a pet, whether it be a dog or a cat, can have numerous benefits for our physical and mental well-being. Studies have shown that pets can reduce stress, anxiety, and depression, and even improve cardiovascular health. Not only do they provide companionship, but caring for a pet can also encourage exercise and playfulness, making it a great option for children and older adults. In fact, pets can even help children grow up to be more secure and active individuals. And perhaps the most special quality of pets is their ability to bring joy and unconditional love into our lives. It's no wonder that they are often considered part of the family.

Multiple studies have shown the numerous physical and mental health benefits of owning a pet. Pet owners are less likely to suffer from depression, have lower blood pressure in stressful situations, and have lower triglyceride and cholesterol levels compared to those without pets. The simple act of playing with a dog or cat can also have a positive impact on our well-being, as it elevates levels of serotonin and dopamine, which promote relaxation. Even more impressive, heart attack patients with pets have been found to survive longer than those without. This may be due to the calming and stress-reducing effects of owning a pet. In fact, pet owners over the age of 65 make 30% fewer visits to their doctors, highlighting the positive impact of pet ownership on overall health. And while dogs and cats are commonly associated with these health benefits, even watching fish in an aquarium can help reduce muscle tension and lower pulse rate. It's clear that owning a pet can greatly improve our physical and mental well-being.

The benefits of pet ownership extend beyond just companionship and love; it has been proven to have therapeutic effects on individuals. One of the reasons for this is that pets fulfil our basic human need for touch, which has been shown to have a calming and soothing effect. Even those who have a history of hardened behaviour, such as criminals in prison, have shown long-term changes in their behaviour after interacting with pets. This interaction allows for the experience of mutual affection, often for the first time. Furthermore, simply stroking, hugging, or touching a loving animal can help to alleviate stress and anxiety. The companionship of a pet can also help to ease feelings of loneliness, and many dogs can serve as a great motivator for healthy exercise, which has been known to boost mood and ease symptoms of depression.

Incorporating a pet into your life can greatly improve your mental health by promoting healthy lifestyle changes. Studies have shown that pets can help ease symptoms of depression, anxiety, stress, bipolar disorder, and PTSD. By taking on the responsibility of caring for a pet, you are forced to establish a routine that includes regular exercise, a healthy diet, and sufficient sleep. This routine can also help to reduce feelings of loneliness and isolation, which are often linked to mental health issues. In addition, pets can provide emotional support and unconditional love, helping to boost self-esteem and reduce negative thoughts and feelings. Overall, adopting a pet can have a positive impact on your mental health by encouraging healthy lifestyle changes and providing much-needed companionship.

Incorporating regular exercise into our daily routines is crucial for both our physical and mental well-being. As dog owners, we have a built-in exercise partner who is always eager to accompany us on walks, hikes, or runs. Not only does this benefit our own health, but studies have shown that dog owners are more likely to meet their daily exercise requirements. Not only that, but regular exercise for our canine companions is also vital for their overall health and behaviour. It can deepen the bond between owner and pet, reduce behaviour problems in dogs, and help keep them physically fit. So let's grab the leash and get moving with our furry exercise buddies!

Studies have shown that providing companionship can have numerous positive effects on our well-being. Caring for a live animal, such as a dog or cat, can give us a sense of purpose and make us feel needed and wanted. This can be especially beneficial for those who live alone, as it can help combat feelings of isolation and loneliness. The act of talking to our pets has also been found to be therapeutic, with many pet owners using their furry friends as a sounding board to work through their troubles. There's nothing quite like the feeling of coming home to a wagging tail or a purring cat to ease the stress of a long day and alleviate feelings of loneliness. By providing companionship, our pets can play a crucial role in improving our overall mental and emotional well-being. Helping you meet new people. Pets can be a great social lubricant for their owners, helping you start and maintain new friendships. Dog owners frequently stop and talk to each other on walks, hikes, or in a dog park. Dog owners also meet new people in pet stores, clubs, and training classes.

Pets can provide much more than just love and entertainment. For people who struggle with anxiety, the companionship of an animal can offer immense comfort and help ease their worries. The unconditional love and non-judgmental nature of pets can make it easier for individuals to go out into the world and face their fears. Furthermore, pets live in the moment and don't worry about the past or future, which can help their owners become more mindful and appreciate the present. By having a furry companion by their side, individuals can build self-confidence and find joy in the simple moments of life. Adding structure and routine to your day. Many pets, especially dogs, require a regular feeding and exercise schedule. Having a consistent routine keeps an animal balanced and calm—and it can work for you, too. No matter your mood—depressed, anxious, or stressed—one plaintive look from your pet and you'll have to get out of bed to feed, exercise, and care for them. Research has shown that touch and movement are effective ways to manage stress in a healthy manner. The simple act of stroking a dog, cat, or other animal has been proven to lower blood pressure and induce a sense of calm and relaxation. In fact, many people turn to their furry companions for sensory stress relief, finding comfort and peace in the soothing touch and movement of their pets. This natural method of stress management can provide quick and effective relief in times of heightened tension, making it a valuable tool for maintaining overall well-being. Whether it's cuddling with a purring cat or taking a walk with a wagging dog, incorporating touch and movement through interactions with animals can greatly improve one's mental and physical state.

13. Hugs

Hugging is a natural and universal way of expressing emotions, from excitement and happiness to sadness and comfort. The act of hugging not only makes us feel good, but it also has proven health benefits. Studies have shown that hugging can lower stress levels and promote a sense of well-being in both the person giving and receiving the hug. So the next time a friend or family member is going through a difficult time, remember the power of a simple hug. By offering support through touch, you can not only provide comfort but also help reduce the stress and burden of the person you care about. And in turn, you may find yourself feeling happier and healthier as well. Let's spread the love and embrace the benefits of hugging.

According to a study conducted on twenty heterosexual couples, researchers found that the act of comforting someone by holding their arm during a distressing event can have a positive impact on our brains. In the study, men were given unpleasant electric shocks while their female partners held their arms. The results showed that the parts of the women's brains associated with stress had reduced activity, while the parts associated with the rewards of maternal behaviour had increased activity. This suggests that the act of hugging someone to comfort them may elicit a similar response in our brains. This research provides valuable insights into the power of human touch and its ability to soothe and comfort during difficult times.

In addition to providing a sense of comfort and connection, hugging may also have health benefits. According to a study of over 400 adults, hugging may reduce the risk of getting sick. Researchers found that individuals with a strong support system, including regular hugs, were less likely to become ill. Even those who did get sick had milder symptoms compared to those with a smaller support system. This suggests that hugging and social support can play a role in boosting the immune system and keeping us healthier. So next time you're feeling stressed or under the weather, consider reaching out for a hug from a loved one. It might just do wonders for your well-being.

According to recent studies, hugging can actually have a positive impact on your heart health. In fact, a study split a group of about 200 adults into two groups and found that the group who engaged in physical touch, such as holding hands for 10 minutes and hugging for 20 seconds, showed greater reductions in blood pressure levels and heart rate compared to the group who simply sat in silence for the same amount of time. This highlights the potential benefits of physical touch and the importance of incorporating it into our relationships and daily lives. So next time you have the opportunity to hug someone you care about, go for it – your heart will thank you! Research has shown that maintaining an affectionate relationship can have positive effects on your heart health. This is due to the presence of oxytocin, also known as the cuddle hormone, in our bodies. Oxytocin levels increase when we engage in physical touch, such as hugging or sitting close to someone, and has been linked to feelings of happiness and reduced stress. Interestingly, studies have found that women may be more affected by oxytocin, as it has been shown to lower blood pressure and the stress hormone norepinephrine. Therefore, it may be beneficial for individuals to prioritize and cultivate close and loving relationships in order to potentially improve their overall heart health.

According to recent research, oxytocin has been found to have the strongest positive effects on women who have close and affectionate relationships with their romantic partners, as well as those who frequently engage in physical touch, such as holding their infants closely. Additionally, studies have shown that touch can significantly reduce anxiety in individuals with low self-esteem, as well as prevent them from isolating themselves when faced with reminders of their mortality. Interestingly, even touching an inanimate object, like a teddy bear, has been found to have a calming effect on individuals and help alleviate fears related to their existence. These findings suggest that the power of touch should not be underestimated, as it can have significant impacts on our well-being and emotional state.

Touch is a powerful form of communication that can have numerous benefits, including reducing pain. Research has shown that therapeutic touch, such as light touching on the skin, can improve quality of life and decrease pain in individuals with fibromyalgia. Hugging is another form of touch that has been found to be beneficial in reducing pain. It is a comforting and communicative way for people to express a range of emotions, including anger, fear, love, and gratitude. In fact, family therapist Virginia Satir once stated that we need at least four hugs a day for survival, eight for maintenance, and 12 for growth. While this may seem like a lot, the positive effects of touch make it clear that more hugs are better than not enough.

In today's society, many people are touch-deprived, which can have negative effects on our overall health and well-being. Despite this, social conventions often discourage touching others, leading to a lack of physical connection and communication. However, studies have shown that regularly hugging and being hugged by loved ones can have a significant impact on our mental and physical health. In fact, it is recommended to have as many hugs as possible each day for optimal benefits. If you feel uncomfortable asking for more hugs, start by seeking them out from your closest friends and family members. Even brief moments of physical connection can positively affect our brains and bodies, leading to reduced stress and improved happiness. So don't be afraid to embrace the power of hugs for a happier and healthier life.

14.Helping others

Scientific studies have shown that when we shift our focus to the needs of others, our stress levels significantly decrease. It's natural for us to get caught up in our own worries and concerns, but taking a moment to redirect our attention towards helping someone else can have a positive impact on our mental and emotional well-being. This is because acts of kindness and selflessness activate the release of oxytocin, a hormone that helps reduce stress and promotes feelings of love and connection. By putting our energy towards others, we are able to find a sense of purpose and fulfilment, leading to a more balanced and healthier state of mind. So the next time you're feeling overwhelmed, try reaching out and lending a helping hand to someone in need. It may just be the stress relief you need.

The power of helping others may have a significant impact on reducing stress and improving overall health, according to a 2015 study published in the Clinical Psychological Science journal. The study, which involved 77 adults aged 18 to 44, found that participants who engaged in acts of kindness reported lower levels of stress and better health outcomes. Each night, the participants received a reminder to complete a daily questionnaire, which helped to track their stress levels and overall well-being. These results highlight the potential benefits of incorporating altruistic acts into our daily lives as a way to combat stress and improve overall health.

A recent study surveyed participants on their daily stressors, including their commute, work, and financial concerns. The questionnaire also tracked their helpful behaviours and acts of kindness, as well as the resulting emotions. The results showed that those who engaged in more acts of kindness on a daily basis were less likely to feel stressed. On days when they were unable to perform any acts of kindness, they reported feeling more stress and negativity. This suggests that by performing small acts of kindness for others, we can effectively manage our own stress levels and improve our overall well-being.

While there is still much to be studied and analysed, this theory shows promising implications for individuals facing high levels of stress. With further research, we can better understand the impact of this theory and potentially utilize it to help those who are struggling. By taking a closer look at the effects of stress and how this theory may play a role in managing it, we can potentially improve the well-being of many individuals. This research could have significant implications for both personal and professional settings, and it is crucial to continue studying this theory in order to fully understand its potential.

Contrary to popular belief, being altruistic doesn't require extreme wealth or an abundance of free time. Even small gestures, such as holding the door open for a stranger, have the potential to reduce stress and bring about positive change. This means that anyone, regardless of their financial status or busy schedule, can reap the benefits of giving back. By incorporating small acts of kindness into our daily lives, we not only make a positive impact on those around us, but also experience a sense of fulfilment and joy within ourselves. So don't underestimate the power of even the smallest acts of altruism – they have the ability to make a big difference in the world.

Here are a few simple deeds you can do to help others and potentially lower your stress levels:

A simple act of kindness can go a long way, and one way to spread positivity and brighten someone's day is by paying it forward at the drive-thru. It may seem like a small gesture, but paying for the car behind you in line can have a big impact on the recipient. Not only will it be a surprise and a pleasant start to their day, but it also requires only a small amount of money. So next time you're in the drive-thru, consider paying it forward and making someone's day a little bit brighter.

Sharing is caring, and this is especially true in the workplace. One easy way to spread kindness and make your colleagues' day a little brighter is by sharing treats in the office break room. Whether you bake a cake or pick up some extra donuts on your way in, your co-workers will appreciate the gesture and enjoy the treat. Additionally, sharing materials like earplugs, tissues, or any other spare items can make a big difference in someone's day. It shows that you are thinking of others and willing to lend a helping hand. So next time you have some extra supplies or treats, consider sharing them with your colleagues. It's a small act of kindness that can go a long way.

De-cluttering our homes not only helps us streamline our living spaces but also provides an opportunity to give back to those in need. One way to do this is by cleaning out our closets or basements and donating old clothes, toys, and books to a nearby shelter. Not only will this help those in need of these goods, but it will also remind us of how fortunate we are to have these items. By clearing out the excess in our lives, we can create a more organized and grateful mindset. So, next time you're cleaning out your closet, consider donating to a local shelter and making a positive impact in both your home and your community.

One impactful way to give back to your community is by volunteering your skills to a local non-profit. Non-profits are always in need of assistance from professionals, whether you are a photographer, web designer, or cook. By volunteering your skills, you can directly contribute to the important work being done by these organizations. Additionally, you can also make a difference by working directly with those in need, such as volunteering at a homeless shelter, animal rescue, or soup kitchen. If you are short on time, you can still make a difference by donating your change to charity when you go grocery shopping or helping in smaller ways like this. Every little bit helps, and your contributions will make a positive impact on those in need and your community as a whole.

At times, it's easy to get caught up in the hustle and bustle of our busy lives and forget about the little things that can make a big difference. That's why it's important to remember to share the love and spread kindness wherever we go. Whether it's a smile, a hug, or a simple squeeze on the shoulder, these gestures may seem small, but they can have a big impact on someone's day. The best part is, they don't require any commitment of time or money. So take a moment to show someone you care, and let them know they have your support. It's the little things that truly make a difference in our relationships and our world.

When it comes to taking care of your health, it's not about big, grand gestures. In fact, it's the small acts of kindness that you do consistently that can make a big difference in your well-being.

Whether it's making healthy food choices every day, taking a walk instead of driving, or simply smiling at a stranger, these small actions can add up over time and have a positive impact on your overall health. So don't underestimate the power of small gestures – they may seem insignificant in the moment, but they can lead to great rewards for your physical and mental well-being.

15. Humour

Laughter truly is the best medicine, providing both mental and physical benefits. From relieving stress to boosting mood, a good laugh has powerful short-term effects. Whether you're watching a sitcom or reading a funny cartoon, laughter can improve your overall well-being. While it may not cure all ailments, there is growing evidence that laughter can have positive impacts on our health. So the next time you feel stressed or down, take a moment to find something to laugh at – your mind and body will thank you.

Laughter can:

Stimulate many organs. Laughter enhances your intake of oxygen-rich air, stimulates your heart, lungs and muscles, and increases the endorphins that are released by your brain.

Activate and relieve your stress response. A rollicking laugh fires up and then cools down your stress response, and it can increase and then decrease your heart rate and blood pressure. The result? A good, relaxed feeling.

Soothe tension. Laughter can also stimulate circulation and aid muscle relaxation, both of which can help reduce some of the physical symptoms of stress.

While we all know that laughter can give us a temporary mood boost, it's important to recognize its long-term benefits as well. Research has shown that laughing can improve our overall health and well-being. It can boost our immune system, decrease stress hormones, and even increase pain tolerance. Plus, laughter is contagious and can strengthen relationships and improve social connections. In the long run, incorporating more laughter into our daily lives can have a positive impact on our mental and physical health. So don't underestimate the power of a good laugh – it's not just a quick fix, but a long-term investment in our well-being.

Laughter may:

Improve your immune system: Negative thoughts manifest into chemical reactions that can affect your body by bringing more stress into your system and decreasing your immunity. By contrast, positive thoughts can actually release neuropeptides that help fight stress and potentially more-serious illnesses.

Relieve pain: Laughter may ease pain by causing the body to produce its own natural painkillers.

Increase personal satisfaction: Laughter can also make it easier to cope with difficult situations. It also helps you connect with other people.

Improve your mood: Many people experience depression, sometimes due to chronic illnesses. Laughter can help lessen your depression and anxiety and may make you feel happier.

Are you afraid you have an underdeveloped — or non-existent — sense of humour? No problem. Humour can be learned. In fact, developing or refining your sense of humour may be easier than you think.

Humour is a powerful tool that can help us navigate through tough times and make everyday life a little brighter. In order to incorporate more humour into your life, it's important to surround yourself with things that make you laugh. This could be as simple as hanging up funny photos or greeting cards at home or in your office. Keeping funny movies, books, or magazines on hand is also a great way to add a little levity to your day. Additionally, exploring joke websites or attending a comedy club can provide a good dose of laughter. So don't be afraid to put humour on your horizon and seek out those simple things that bring a smile to your face.

It's often said that laughter is the best medicine, and when it comes to managing stress, this statement holds true. When we find ways to laugh, whether it's through finding humour in our own situations or trying laughter yoga, we can see our stress levels decrease. It may feel awkward or forced at first, but practicing laughter can do wonders for our physical and mental health. Laughter yoga, where groups come together to practice laughter, is a great way to start. Even if it starts out as forced laughter, it can quickly turn into genuine laughter and help us let go of stress. So go ahead and give it a try, because as they say, laughter is contagious.

It's important to make time for laughter in our lives. Whether it's spending time with friends who always make us laugh or sharing funny stories and jokes with those around us, laughter can bring joy and positivity into our lives. Not only does it make us feel good, but it also strengthens our relationships with others. So make it a habit to surround yourself with people who bring laughter and joy into your life, and don't be afraid to spread the love by sharing funny moments and jokes with those around you. Remember, laughter is the best medicine and can help improve our overall well-being.

Humour is an essential part of life, and one way to bring some joy into our daily routines is through jokes. Whether it's a classic knock-knock joke or a witty one-liner, jokes can bring a smile to anyone's face. Next time you're at your local bookstore or library, take a moment to browse through their selection of joke books and add a few jokes to your list. Then, you can share them with your friends and spread some laughter. With so much negativity in the world, it's important to take a moment to appreciate the power of a good joke and its ability to bring people together. So go ahead, knock, knock, and add some humour to your day.

Humour is a powerful tool, but it's important to know when it's appropriate and when it's not. Laughing at the expense of others or using humour that is hurtful or inappropriate is never okay. It's important to use our best judgment to discern what is a good joke and what is not. If you have any doubts about a joke, it's best to err on the side of caution and avoid it. Humour should bring people together, not divide them. So let's make sure to use humour responsibly and thoughtfully, and always keep in mind the impact our words can have on others.

In today's fast-paced and often stressful work environments, taking a moment to laugh can do wonders for our mental and physical well-being. So why not give it a try? It may feel a bit forced at first, but turning the corners of your mouth up into a smile and giving a little laugh can help to release tension in your muscles and leave you feeling more relaxed and light-hearted. This simple act can be especially beneficial during busy and hectic workdays, allowing us to reset and refocus on the tasks at hand. So don't be afraid to embrace the natural wonder of laughing at work – your mind and body will thank you for it.

16. Gratitude

Maintaining a positive attitude is a valuable skill that can greatly benefit our lives, especially during challenging times. While it may seem like some people are naturally inclined to have a positive outlook, the truth is that anyone can cultivate this mindset with practice. It's about shifting our perspective and focusing on the good in difficult situations and people. By appreciating what we have, even in the face of loss, we can increase our ability to maintain a positive attitude and handle stress more effectively. With determination and dedication, we can all learn to see the good in life and maintain a positive mindset, no matter what comes our way.

Luckily, developing a positive attitude is possible with consistent effort. While we may have natural inclinations towards certain temperaments, our brains are like muscles and can be strengthened towards optimism. The good news is that working on our gratitude muscle can actually be an enjoyable process. And the best part is that the benefits we gain from this effort make it well worth it, even if it may seem like a challenging task at first.

Research has shown that building emotional resilience and maintaining a positive outlook can greatly improve overall well-being. One key factor in achieving this is practicing gratitude. By actively cultivating a sense of gratitude, individuals can experience a more positive mood in their daily lives and reap social benefits as well. This practice has been found to contribute to greater emotional well-being, making it an essential tool for those seeking to enhance their overall quality of life. So why not start incorporating gratitude into your daily routine and see the positive impact it can have on your emotional resilience and optimism?

Cultivating gratitude can have a profound impact on our overall well-being and happiness. Research has shown that individuals who actively practice gratitude tend to experience higher levels of emotional well-being and life satisfaction. Grateful individuals also tend to have stronger and more fulfilling relationships, as they are more appreciative of their loved ones. This appreciation can create a positive cycle, as loved ones often reciprocate and do more to earn it. Furthermore, the positive effects of gratitude can also extend to our physical health, as those who are happier and have healthier relationships also tend to have better sleep and overall health. By actively practicing gratitude, we can improve our quality of life and foster a more positive outlook.

In our busy lives, it's easy to get caught up in negative thoughts and stressors, leaving little room for feelings of gratitude. However, the good news is that gratitude can be developed through various exercises. Over the next few weeks, try incorporating some of these activities into your daily routine. Not only will you begin to notice more positive aspects of your life, but you may also find yourself dwelling less on negative events and feelings of lack. Ultimately, you will cultivate a deeper sense of appreciation for the people and things in your life. So take the time to nurture gratitude, and you'll reap the benefits in your overall well-being.

In times of stress or when faced with negative events, it can be easy to get caught up in our complaints and grievances. However, a powerful tool for shifting our mindset and finding peace is to actively practice gratitude. Instead of focusing on the negative, try to think of four or five things that you are grateful for in that same situation. For example, when feeling overwhelmed at work, remind yourself of the aspects of your job that you enjoy and appreciate. The same can be done for relationship stress, financial difficulties, or daily annoyances. By gently reminding ourselves of the positives, we can begin to shift our perspective and find gratitude in even the most challenging situations. With practice, this can become a powerful tool for finding peace and happiness in our daily lives.

In today's world of social media, it's easy to fall into the trap of making comparisons to others and feeling inadequate. However, this can cause unnecessary stress and hinder our ability to feel gratitude. It's important to remember that we often compare ourselves to those who seem to have more, do more, or are closer to our ideals. Instead, we can choose to shift our perspective and compare ourselves to those who have less, reminding ourselves of how truly fortunate we are. Additionally, we can also choose to feel grateful for the people in our lives who inspire us, rather than letting comparison lead to envy. By choosing either of these paths, we can reduce the stress and negativity caused by social comparison and cultivate a mindset of gratitude.

A simple and effective way to cultivate gratitude in your daily life is to start a gratitude journal. By combining the benefits of journaling with the active practice of focusing on the positive aspects of your life, you can create a catalogue of happy memories and a long list of things you are grateful for. This can be especially helpful during times when it may be difficult to remember these things. By consistently writing in your gratitude journal for two to three weeks, you can form a habit that will require less and less effort to maintain over time. This will result in a more positive and less stress-inducing attitude becoming automatic for you, leading to greater feelings of emotional well-being.

17. Crying

Crying is a natural and universal human action, often triggered by a wide range of emotions. But beyond just being a form of emotional expression, research has shown that crying can actually have several health benefits for both the body and the mind. In fact, these benefits can begin as early as a baby's first cry. According to studies, crying can help release toxins and relieve stress by lowering our levels of cortisol, the hormone associated with stress. Additionally, tears contain lysozyme, an enzyme that can help fight off bacteria and keep our eyes clean and healthy. Furthermore, crying can also provide emotional release and help us process and cope with difficult emotions. So next time you feel the urge to cry, don't hold back - it may be beneficial for your overall well-being.

There are three different types of tears:

1. reflex tears
2. continuous tears
3. emotional tears

As a complex and important bodily function, tears serve a variety of purposes for our eyes. Reflex tears are responsible for clearing debris, such as smoke and dust, from our eyes to maintain clear vision. Meanwhile, continuous tears work to lubricate and protect our eyes from potential infections. Interestingly, emotional tears contain not only water but also stress hormones and other toxins. Some researchers have proposed that crying may serve as a way to flush these substances out of our bodies, but more studies are needed to fully understand the potential health benefits of emotional tears. Regardless, it's clear that tears play a crucial role in maintaining the health and function of our eyes.

Crying can often be seen as a sign of weakness or vulnerability, but research shows that it may actually be a helpful mechanism for self-soothing. Studies have found that crying triggers the parasympathetic nervous system (PNS), which helps our bodies rest and digest. Although the benefits of crying may not be immediate, as it can take several minutes of shedding tears to feel the soothing effects, it can ultimately be a beneficial way to cope with emotions and find comfort. So next time you feel the urge to cry, don't hold back, as it may be just what your body needs to calm down and relax.

Crying is a natural and healthy way to cope with emotional and physical pain. When we cry for extended periods of time, our bodies release oxytocin and endorphins, also known as feel-good chemicals. These chemicals can help ease both physical and emotional pain, and may even lead to a sense of calm or well-being. This is why crying is often seen as a self-soothing action. The release of endorphins can also cause a numbing effect, helping us to temporarily disconnect from our emotions and find some relief. So next time you find yourself in tears, remember that it's a normal and beneficial way to cope with pain.

Crying, specifically sobbing, can have surprising benefits beyond simply releasing pent-up emotions. Along with helping to ease pain, sobbing can also lift your spirits. This is because when you sob, you take in many quick breaths of cool air, which helps to regulate and lower the temperature of your brain. A cooler brain can be more pleasurable to both your body and mind, potentially leading to an improvement in mood after a sobbing episode. So the next time you feel overwhelmed with emotion, don't be afraid to let it out and embrace a good sob. Your body and mind may thank you for it. Top of Form

Bottom of Form

If you're feeling blue, crying is a way to let those around you know you are in need of support. This is known as an interpersonal benefit. From the time you were a baby, crying has been an attachment behaviour. Its function is in many ways to obtain comfort and care from others. In other words, it helps to build up your social support network when the going gets tough.

Grieving is a natural and necessary process that occurs when we experience a loss. It is not a linear process and involves a range of emotions, including sorrow, numbness, guilt, and anger. One important aspect of grieving is allowing yourself to cry. Crying can be a cathartic release and can help you process and accept the loss of a loved one. It is a way for your body to release built-up emotions and can be a sign of healthy coping. While it may be difficult and uncomfortable, allowing yourself to cry is an important step in the grieving process. It is important to remember that there is no right or wrong way to grieve and everyone experiences it differently. Be gentle with yourself and allow yourself to feel and express your emotions in whatever way feels right to you.

It's important to remember that the grieving process is unique for each individual. While crying is a natural response to grief, if it becomes excessive or begins to disrupt your daily routine, it may be beneficial to consult with a medical professional. It's also worth noting that crying is not limited to just sadness; it can also occur in moments of extreme joy, fear, or stress. In fact, researchers at Yale University suggest that crying in these instances can help restore emotional balance. When we experience intense emotions and cry, it may be our body's way of processing and recovering from such strong feelings. So if you find yourself crying in moments of happiness or fear, know that it is a normal and healthy response. However, if you feel like your crying is excessive or interfering with your well-being, seeking medical advice may be helpful.

18. Fun

As adults, we often get caught up in the never-ending cycle of responsibilities and obligations. The thought of incorporating fun activities into our lives can feel like a luxury we can't afford. However, making time for fun can actually be one of the best stress relief tips to follow. We may have adult-sized responsibilities, but neglecting our inner child can lead to feelings of stagnation and unhappiness. By taking the time to let loose and have fun, we can feel more alive and rejuvenated. Not only that, but there are numerous benefits to having good old fun, such as increased creativity, improved relationships, and a better overall sense of well-being. So why not make a conscious effort to prioritize fun in your life? You may be surprised at how much better you feel when you allow yourself to let go and have some fun.

Engaging in fun activities is crucial for our overall well-being, as it provides a source of eustress, also known as the 'good' kind of stress. This type of stress helps us feel invigorated and energized, and it's the feeling of excitement that comes from completing a project, riding a roller coaster, or tackling a challenging task. It's essential to have a healthy balance of eustress in our lives, and participating in fun activities is a great way to achieve that. Whether it's trying a new hobby, taking a trip, or simply spending time with loved ones, these activities can provide the necessary dose of eustress to keep us feeling vital and alive. So make sure to prioritize fun and enjoyable activities in your life to maintain a healthy and balanced mindset.

In today's fast-paced and high-pressure world, stress has become a constant companion for many of us. However, incorporating regular moments of fun into our lives can help alleviate some of the overwhelming feelings that come with stress. By finding joy in the small things and making time for activities we enjoy, we can change our attitude towards the stressors in our lives. This, in turn, can make us less reactive when faced with stressful situations. So don't forget to take a break, have some fun, and prioritize your mental and emotional well-being.

In addition to boosting our mood and overall well-being, laughter has numerous health benefits. From reducing stress and anxiety to strengthening our immune system, incorporating more laughter into our daily lives can have a significant impact on our health. While it may be challenging to find time to hit the gym or resist unhealthy comfort foods when we're feeling stressed, making room for fun and laughter is something that is both beneficial and easily attainable. So go ahead and add some more laughter to your day, your mind and body will thank you for it!

One of the keys to a healthy and fulfilling relationship is constantly finding new ways to connect and have fun together. When couples make an effort to engage in new activities and experiences together, it can strengthen their bond and prevent them from falling into a rut. Not only does this bring excitement and joy into the relationship, but it also serves as a great source of stress relief in our busy lives. Making time for each other and prioritizing shared experiences can ultimately lead to a closer and more fulfilling relationship. So, next time you and your partner are feeling overwhelmed, consider trying something new together as a way to reconnect and de-stress.

Just as spending time with friends can help maintain a supportive circle and decrease stress levels, cultivating strong professional relationships can also have a positive impact on our overall well-being. Research has shown that having a sense of community and strong friendships in the workplace can lead to increased longevity, lower stress levels, and improved health. This is why it's important to not only focus on our individual work tasks, but also take the time to connect with our colleagues and build a supportive network. By fostering positive professional relationships, we can create a more positive and healthy work environment for ourselves and our team.

In the midst of a demanding job with high expectations and little recognition, it's important to have activities that can help prevent burnout. Regularly engaging in fun and rewarding activities is a great way to relieve stress and boost morale. These activities can include giving yourself small rewards or forming a support group with friends to celebrate accomplishments that may otherwise go unnoticed. By making time for fun and surrounding yourself with a positive community, you can combat the negative effects of burnout and maintain a healthy work-life balance.

19. Singing

The benefits of singing extend beyond just improving vocal skills or expressing oneself artistically. In fact, research conducted at the University of Frankfurt has shown that singing can actually boost the immune system. The study involved testing professional choir members' blood before and after an hour-long rehearsal of Mozart's Requiem. The results showed that after singing, the levels of Immunoglobulin A, which are proteins that act as antibodies in the immune system, were significantly higher. This increase was not seen when the choir members passively listened to music, highlighting the unique impact that singing has on the body. So, not only is singing a fun and enjoyable activity, but it may also have important health benefits as well.

Singing is a form of exercise that offers a wide range of benefits for individuals of all ages and abilities. For the elderly, disabled, and injured, it can provide a low-impact form of physical activity that promotes improved lung function and circulation. Even for those who are in good health, singing can still offer a workout for the diaphragm and increased oxygen intake, leading to improved aerobic capacity and stamina. By using proper singing techniques and vocal projections, individuals can reap the numerous health benefits that come with this enjoyable form of exercise. So whether you're looking to maintain your health or improve it, consider incorporating singing into your regular routine.

In the world of singing, proper technique is crucial for both vocal health and performance. This includes standing up straight with good posture. Over time, practicing good posture while singing will become a habit, allowing you to effortlessly maintain proper form. As you align your shoulders and back and expand your chest cavity while singing, you are also improving your posture in general. This not only benefits your vocal abilities, but also your overall physical well-being. So remember, always stand tall and straight while singing for the best results!

In a recent article published by Daily Mail Online, health experts revealed that singing may actually have a positive impact on snoring and sleep apnoea. This is because singing exercises and strengthens the muscles in the throat and palate, which can help alleviate these common sleep problems. For those who struggle with snoring or sleep apnoea, this news may come as a relief as getting a good night's sleep can be a difficult feat. So next time you're belting out your favourite tunes, remember that you're not just entertaining yourself, but also potentially improving your sleep quality.

Not only does singing bring joy to our lives, but it also has a physiological impact on our brains. As we sing, our bodies release endorphins, which are the feel-good chemicals that promote feelings of happiness and well-being. Scientists have also discovered that the sacculus, a tiny organ in the ear, responds to the frequencies created by singing, resulting in an immediate sense of pleasure. It doesn't matter how good or bad we may sound; the act of singing alone can lift our spirits. Furthermore, singing can serve as a distraction from the stresses of daily life, providing a much-needed boost to our mood. So, whether you're a trained vocalist or simply love belting out your favourite tunes in the shower, keep on singing for your mental and emotional well-being.

The act of making music in any form can be a highly effective way to relax and reduce stress. Not only does singing release tension in the muscles, but it also decreases the levels of cortisol, a stress hormone, in the body. The physical benefits of singing also extend to improved blood circulation and oxygenation, allowing more oxygen to reach the brain. This, in turn, can improve mental alertness, concentration, and memory. In fact, the Alzheimer's Society has even recognized the therapeutic benefits of singing and offers a Singing for the Brain service to help individuals with dementia and Alzheimer's maintain their memories. So whether you're a professional singer or just enjoy belting out tunes in the shower, making music can have a positive impact on both your physical and mental well-being.

In addition to the joy and pleasure that comes from singing, it also offers unexpected health benefits that can enhance your social life. Whether you are a member of a choir or simply enjoy belting out tunes with friends at karaoke, singing can foster deep bonds with others due to the inherent intimacy involved. Although it's common for new singers to experience stage fright, receiving praise from loved ones and performing well can help to overcome these fears and build self-confidence. With continued practice and experience, you may find it easier to present any type of material in front of a group with poise and excellent presentation skills. So, don't be afraid to share your love for singing with others and reap the many benefits it can bring to your social life.

As The Guardian suggests, singing to babies can have a significant impact on their language development. It is just as crucial as teaching reading and writing at a young age to prevent language problems later in life. This means that parents and caregivers should not underestimate the power of music in their child's early education. In fact, honing one's own lyrical abilities can improve their communication skills in various ways. So don't be afraid to break out into song with your little one, as it could greatly benefit their future language abilities.

As we progress and improve in our skills, we often seek inspiration and guidance from those who have mastered their craft. It's a natural part of growth, and we may even discover new styles and techniques that we would not have appreciated before. It's important to remember that the journey of improvement is ongoing, and there will always be new challenges and lessons to learn. But by looking to the masters and expanding our horizons, we can continue to push ourselves and reach new levels of skill and creativity. So don't be afraid to step out of your comfort zone and try new things – you never know what you might discover.

Singing is not only a delightful activity but also offers numerous health benefits that may encourage you to take up the hobby. Not only does it allow you to appreciate the beauty of your own vocal talent, but it also helps improve lung capacity, reduce stress levels, and boost your immune system. These benefits are so significant that you may feel inclined to join a choir or start taking voice lessons right away. Don't hesitate to do so and have fun with it. Remember, it's important to do what you enjoy and what makes you happy. So if singing is something you love, don't hold back and let your voice shine!

20. Sport

The benefits of regular exercise are well-documented and include weight loss, increased strength, and improved overall health. However, in addition to physical benefits, exercise has also been shown to have a positive impact on mental health. In times of anxiety, engaging in physical activity can be an effective way to ease the mind. Exercise releases endorphins, also known as feel-good hormones, which can help reduce stress and improve mood. So not only is exercise beneficial for your physical health, but it can also be a powerful tool for maintaining mental wellness. Make sure to incorporate regular exercise into your routine to reap all of these benefits for both your body and mind.

One of the great things about exercise is that it can boost our mood by increasing the production of endorphins in our body. And the best part? Any type of physical activity can provide these benefits. From taking a leisurely walk or bike ride to practicing yoga or trying out a new workout, simply moving our bodies can have a positive impact on our mental well-being. So don't feel limited to a certain type of exercise, just find what works for you and enjoy the benefits it brings.

Incorporating exercise into your daily routine can have numerous benefits, including improving your sleep quality. If you're feeling stressed and haven't been physically active, why not give sports a try? You don't have to aim for the tennis world champion title, just start by getting your body moving. You'll likely feel the benefits after your very first time playing. And once you experience the positive effects of exercise, you won't want to go back to a sedentary lifestyle filled with stress. So go ahead and give it a try, your body and mind will thank you.

In today's busy world, it's not always easy to find the time or motivation to get active. Whether you're not a fan of sweating it out or simply don't have the time, there are still ways to reap the stress-relieving benefits of sports. You may find that tuning into some sports action on TV is just what you need. Research has shown that even just watching sports can help lower stress levels, making it a great option for those who prefer a more low-key approach. So, next time you're feeling overwhelmed, grab the remote and tune in to your favourite team or event for a dose of stress relief.

Finding a sport to watch and enjoy can be a great way to unwind after a long and stressful day. Whether you prefer the intensity of an Olympic qualifier, the excitement of a Champions League football match, or the thrill of following NCAAF lines, immersing yourself in a sport can help you relax and take your mind off any worries or stress. With so many sports to choose from, there is something for everyone to enjoy and find solace in, making it a perfect activity for unwinding and taking it easy. So go ahead and pick your favourite sport to watch, and let yourself relax and enjoy the excitement and thrill it brings.

It's important to recognize that stress can often be accompanied by feelings of loneliness or isolation. These emotions can be especially difficult to manage when you have no one to talk to or turn to for support. However, finding a common interest, such as a love for sports, can help bridge that gap and bring people together. Whether it's striking up a conversation with someone at the gym or joining a sports team, participating in physical activities can help foster connections and alleviate feelings of isolation. Even something as simple as going for a bike ride or joining a local walking or climbing group can lead to new friendships and a sense of belonging. So don't underestimate the power of shared interests when it comes to combating stress and loneliness.

The sense of community and camaraderie at a sports stadium is unparalleled. It's not uncommon to strike up a conversation with a stranger sitting beside you and find a common passion for the game. The same goes for a sports bar, where you can easily make new friends who share your interests. Whether you're at the stadium or the bar, the shared experience of cheering on your team creates a sense of belonging and brings people together in a powerful way. So next time you attend a game, don't be afraid to strike up a conversation with your fellow spectators – you never know, you may just make a new friend!

Sports have been proven to have a positive impact on one's overall well-being. Not only can they provide a much-needed break from the stresses of daily life, but they also offer a way to improve physical health and mental clarity. Engaging in sports allows for an outlet to release tension and frustration, leading to a more relaxed and positive mindset. In addition, the social aspect of sports can foster connections and a sense of community, which can further contribute to a happier and healthier life. If you're looking to reduce stress and improve your overall well-being, incorporating sports into your routine is a great place to start.

21. Jogging

The benefits of jogging and running go far beyond just physical health. In fact, there are numerous psychological benefits that can greatly improve one's overall well-being. Not only does this type of aerobic exercise increase mental flexibility and clarity, but it also boosts confidence and serves as a form of stress relief. Furthermore, the release of natural mood-elevating compounds can lead to a sense of emotional well-being commonly known as the runner's high. The challenges and perseverance required in running can also teach valuable lessons about oneself that can be applied to other areas of life. Overall, incorporating jogging or running into one's fitness routine can have a positive impact on both physical and mental health.

Aside from the physical benefits, running also has a profound impact on the mind. Through running, individuals learn to cultivate focus and determination, allowing them to overcome obstacles and fatigue. It provides a new perspective on both large and small problems, showing individuals their true capabilities and inner strength to endure and conquer challenges. The willpower and resilience that helps a runner push through a long run or motivate themselves to get out the door on a day when they'd rather stay in bed are the same qualities that give them strength in other aspects of life. Running is not just a physical exercise, but a powerful mental training as well.

There's no denying the transformative power of running. As an individual sport, it allows you to push yourself, conquer challenges, and emerge stronger and more confident with each stride. It's a constant battle against trials and obstacles, and each victory fuels a sense of empowerment and freedom. With each step, you build not only physical strength but also mental resilience, proving to yourself that your body is capable of achieving great things. So lace up your shoes and hit the pavement, because the confidence you'll gain from running is unlike any other.

According to recent research, engaging in physical activities such as running and jogging can have a direct impact on one's self-esteem. By consistently participating in exercise, individuals reported feeling better about their overall fitness level and body image, both of which were strongly connected to improved self-esteem. This finding highlights the importance of regular physical activity not only for physical health, but also for mental and emotional well-being. It is clear that taking care of our bodies through exercise can have a positive impact on how we feel about ourselves, leading to improved self-esteem and overall satisfaction with our bodies.

Aside from the physical benefits, running or jogging also provides valuable stress relief. Not only does it offer a temporary escape from daily troubles, but research shows that sticking to a consistent running routine can lead to long-term stress relief benefits. By incorporating running into your self-care routine, you can build resilience and improve your ability to handle life's challenges. This is because regular exercise has been linked to increased levels of endorphins, the feel-good hormones, and can help reduce the levels of stress hormones in the body. So lace up your sneakers and hit the pavement for a healthy dose of stress relief.

Aside from the physical benefits of running, it also has a significant impact on our mental health. The well-known runner's high is a real phenomenon that triggers feelings of happiness and can reduce stress levels. This is because running stimulates the release of endorphins in our bodies, leading to a sense of euphoria. In fact, studies have shown that a long-distance run can increase opioid binding in various areas of the brain, further enhancing these positive emotions. So not only does running benefit our physical well-being, but it also has a positive effect on our mental well-being.

The benefits of running and jogging go beyond just physical fitness. In fact, these activities can have a positive impact on your overall attitude and well-being. The release of endorphins during a run can result in a feeling of happiness and well-being, which can have a significant impact on your mood and outlook on life. Whether it's a quick burst of well-being or a general sense of happiness, the positive influences of running and jogging on your attitude can help you manage and relieve daily stress. So next time you lace up your running shoes, remember that you're not just improving your physical health, but also your mental and emotional well-being.

It's no secret that regular exercise has numerous benefits for both physical and mental health. In fact, research has shown that engaging in exercise, such as running, can have a positive impact on mood and anxiety disorders. A study conducted in 2013 found that exercise was more effective than no therapy in reducing depressive symptoms. However, it's worth noting that the study also found that exercise was not significantly more effective than antidepressants. Despite this, incorporating regular exercise into one's routine can still have significant benefits for managing and improving symptoms of mood and anxiety disorders. It's important to consult with a healthcare professional to determine the best course of treatment for each individual case.

Patients who have incorporated a regular running program into their treatment have experienced significant improvements in their mental health. The physical act of running has been shown to reduce tension, depression, fatigue, and confusion, among other symptoms. This form of exercise provides patients with a healthy outlet to focus on, allowing them to shift their attention away from their depressed state or addiction. By incorporating running into their daily routine, patients have seen a positive impact on their overall well-being and mental   state.

22. Hit the gym

Even on the most challenging days, it's important to prioritize self-care. While it may be tempting to retreat into the comfort of your own home, hitting the gym for a workout can have numerous benefits. Not only does exercise improve your physical health, but it can also help alleviate stress and improve your overall well-being. So, instead of giving in to the urge to hibernate, consider heading to the gym for an invigorating workout that will leave you feeling refreshed and rejuvenated. The calming effects of physical activity can work wonders on melting away the tension and frustrations of a difficult day, leaving you feeling ready to take on whatever comes your way. Don't underestimate the power of self-care, even on the toughest of days.

Regular exercise has numerous physical benefits, but did you know it can also boost your mood? It's no coincidence that you feel a sense of joy and happiness after a workout. This is because exercise causes the release of endorphins in your brain, which are neurotransmitters that can elevate your mood. It doesn't matter what type of exercise you do – whether it's running on a treadmill or dancing in a Zumba class – you'll still experience the same elevated mood. This is commonly referred to as a runner's high, but it can happen with any form of physical activity. So next time you're feeling down, consider going for a jog or attending a fitness class to boost your mood and reap the physical and mental benefits of exercise.

Meditation

Engaging in physical activity is not only beneficial for our physical health, but it can also have a positive impact on our mental well-being. By concentrating on our chosen exercise, we can enter a meditative-like state that allows us to let go of any stress or distractions. Whether it's focusing on our breathing rhythm while running on a treadmill or feeling our feet hitting the pavement while taking a jog outside, these specific actions can help clear our minds and alleviate our stress levels. So the next time you feel overwhelmed or stressed, consider taking a break and engaging in some physical activity to find a sense of peace and relaxation.

Social Exercises

For many individuals, going to the gym is not just about working out, but also about connecting with others. Whether it's with friends or family members, taking a yoga, step aerobics, or dance class together can provide a social outlet that helps alleviate the stresses of the day. Joining a gym can also expand your social circle, potentially leading to new friendships that can greatly enhance your life. According to MayoClinic.com, exercising with a partner can increase your commitment to physical activity, making it more likely that you'll stick with it and see the results you desire. So next time you hit the gym, don't be afraid to strike up a conversation with your workout buddy – it could lead to a stronger body and a stronger social circle.

It's no secret that being unhappy with our bodies can cause a great deal of stress and anxiety. However, there is a solution that not only improves our physical health, but also boosts our self-esteem: working out. Whether you struggle with dating due to your weight or have unhealthy habits such as drinking and smoking, regularly visiting the gym can help you shed pounds and develop a healthier lifestyle. According to MayoClinic.com, exercise can also lead to a sense of calmness through the increase in body temperature. By incorporating exercise into your routine, you can not only improve your physical health, but also your mental and emotional well-being.

23.   Dancing

It's no secret that dancing can be a great stress reliever, and this is precisely why Kevin Bacon's iconic dance scene in Footloose resonates with so many of us. As teenagers, we often carry a lot of drama and stress, and dancing provides a cathartic outlet to release these pent-up emotions. It's no wonder that at prom, where we're finally given the opportunity to let loose and dance, we feel a sense of freedom and release. So next time you're feeling overwhelmed or anxious, why not put on some music and dance it out? It might just be the perfect stress-relieving activity for you.

What is it about dancing that makes us all feel so free and relieved of our everyday stresses?

There is a scientific explanation for the stress-relieving effects of dance. When we engage in physical activity, our bodies release neurotransmitters and endorphins, which are responsible for improving our mood and reducing stress. Neurotransmitters act as messengers in the brain, while endorphins act as natural painkillers. Together, they work to promote a sense of calm and optimism in the body. This also leads to improved sleep quality, which can help prevent sleepless nights caused by stress. So, next time you're feeling overwhelmed, consider taking a dance break to boost your mood and reduce stress. Your mind and body will thank you.

In the professional world, it can often feel like you have to conform and hide your true self in order to fit in and succeed. This can be exhausting and lead to a sense of disconnection from who we really are. However, dancing offers a much-needed outlet for self-expression, whether it's through the music, movement, or even costumes. It allows us to let go of the pressures of our work environment and truly connect with our inner selves. So why not leave behind the suit and pencil skirt and trade them in for some sparkles and spandex? Dancing can be a powerful tool for embracing and celebrating who we truly are, without the restrictions of our professional personas.

Dancing is not just a fun activity, but it's also a total body workout with a wide range of benefits. Whether you're looking to lose weight, improve flexibility, strengthen your bones, or build muscle tone, dancing has got you covered. It's a form of exercise that engages the entire body, from head to toe, making it a great option for overall fitness. Plus, with a variety of dance styles to choose from, there's something for everyone to enjoy and reap the benefits from. So next time you're looking for a way to get in shape, consider adding some dance moves into your routine for a well-rounded and enjoyable workout.

Dancing can be a way to stay fit for people of all ages, shapes and sizes. It has a wide range of physical and mental benefits including:

1. Improved condition of your heart and lungs
2. Increased muscular strength, endurance and motor fitness
3. Increased aerobic fitness
4. Improved muscle tone and strength
Weight management
5. Stronger bones and reduced risk of osteoporosis
6. Better coordination, agility and flexibility
7. Improved balance and spatial awareness
8. Increased physical confidence
9. Improved mental functioning
10. Improved general and psychological well being
11. Greater self-confidence and self-esteem
12. Better social skills.

Prioritizing our health and wellness is essential for leading a fulfilling and stress-free life. Taking care of ourselves physically and mentally should always be a top priority, as it allows us to function at our best and tackle life's challenges with a clear and focused mind. Engaging in activities that promote our well-being, such as exercise, healthy eating, and self-care practices, can have a significant impact on our overall happiness and stress levels. So let's make a conscious effort to prioritize our health and make it a regular part of our routine, because there's nothing more satisfying than knowing we're doing something positive for our well-being.

In our fast-paced and hectic world, it's no secret that stress can have detrimental effects on our physical and mental well-being. From increased inflammation in the heart to psychological distress, stress has been dubbed as a silent killer. However, there is a simple and enjoyable way to combat and prevent these negative effects:

dancing. Just like the iconic Footloose crew, we can let loose and dance our stress away. So next time you're feeling overwhelmed, take a cue from Kevin Bacon and dance it out!

24. Sound Healing

Sound healing is a well-established practice that utilizes the power of sound and vibration to improve our physical and mental well-being. Despite its seemingly mystical nature, sound healing is firmly rooted in scientific principles. By utilizing different sound frequencies, we can influence our brainwaves and physiological processes, leading to reduced stress, improved sleep, and overall better health. This therapy has gained popularity in recent years, and its effectiveness has been supported by numerous studies. So, whether you're looking to reduce anxiety, enhance creativity, or simply relax, sound healing may be just the solution you need.

Sound healing is based on the belief that everything in our world, including our own bodies, is in a state of constant vibration. From our cells and tissues to our organs, each part of our being has its own unique frequency. However, when we encounter stress or illness, these frequencies can become disrupted or imbalanced. Sound healing aims to restore and rebalance these vibrations, using the power of sound and vibration to promote relaxation, reduce stress, and improve overall well-being. By harnessing the healing properties of sound, this practice offers a holistic approach to healing and wellness.

The practice of sound healing aims to restore harmony and balance within the body by exposing it to specific sound frequencies. This approach is rooted in the concept of resonance, where one vibrating object can influence another object to vibrate at the same frequency. This phenomenon is often demonstrated by an opera singer shattering a glass with their voice at its resonant frequency. Similarly, within the human body, different parts have their own unique resonant frequencies. By utilizing sound healing techniques, it is believed that these frequencies can be brought into alignment, promoting overall wellness and well-being. This holistic approach to healing has gained popularity in recent years and is used by many to address a variety of physical and emotional ailments.

The Role of Meditation in Sound Healing for Stress Reduction

As individuals, we are constantly faced with stressors in our daily lives, from work pressures to personal obligations. While meditation has long been recognized as a powerful tool for reducing stress, combining it with sound healing can enhance its effects even further. By incorporating sound therapy, such as the use of singing bowls or chanting, into your meditation practice, you can achieve a deeper state of relaxation and release tension from both the mind and body. The combination of these two techniques can help to alleviate stress and promote overall well-being. By integrating meditation with sound healing, you can create a more comprehensive and effective stress relief practice for yourself.

Incorporating sound healing into guided meditation sessions can greatly enhance the experience and benefits of this practice. By using elements such as singing bowls, chimes, or binaural beats, the soothing tones can help deepen relaxation and create a more immersive experience. A meditation guide or recording will lead participants through a calming journey, focusing on the breath, visualizing peaceful scenes, and listening to the accompanying sounds. This combination of mindfulness and sound healing can be especially effective for reducing stress and promoting overall well-being.

For those who prefer a self-guided approach, incorporating sound healing into your meditation routine can be a powerful and effective way to relax and release tension. Begin by finding a quiet and uninterrupted space, allowing yourself to fully immerse in the experience. Choose your preferred sound healing instrument or audio recording, whether it be a singing bowl, chimes, or a guided meditation with sound elements. Close your eyes and take deep breaths, allowing the soothing sounds to guide you into a state of relaxation. As you focus on your breath and the sounds around you, you can also focus on releasing tension and stress with each exhale. With a self-guided meditation, you have the freedom to create a routine that works best for you and your specific needs.

25. Punch bag

The benefits of boxing as an exercise are vast and often overlooked. This physically and mentally demanding sport offers a wide range of health benefits, making it a popular choice for those looking to improve their overall well-being. From improving cardiovascular health and strength to relieving stress and boosting confidence, boxing has much more to offer than many people realize. It's a versatile form of exercise that can be tailored to fit your specific goals, whether you aspire to become a professional boxer or simply want a challenging cardio workout. The results of incorporating boxing into your fitness routine are consistent and proven, making it a worthy pursuit for anyone looking to improve their health and wellness.

Aside from the physical advantages, it's important to recognize the positive impact boxing can have on your mental health. It's not just about fighting others, but rather the entire process of training and perfecting your skills in the ring. From improving your stamina to honing your technique, every aspect of boxing can have a lasting and meaningful effect on your overall well-being. The discipline, focus, and confidence gained from boxing can extend beyond the ring and positively impact other areas of your life as well. So don't underestimate the power of this sport for both your physical and mental health.

Regular exercise has been scientifically linked to improved mental health, making it an essential part of any wellness routine. By engaging in physical activity, the body releases endorphins, chemicals that promote a sense of happiness and well-being. This natural boost in mood can be a great way to combat stress, anxiety, and other mental health issues. Whether it's going for a run, lifting weights, or even just taking a brisk walk, any form of exercise can have a positive impact on your overall well-being. So don't hesitate to incorporate physical activity into your daily routine to reap the benefits for both your physical and mental health.

In addition to the immediate benefits of exercise, such as improved mood and energy levels, incorporating regular physical activity into your daily routine can also have long-term benefits. By consistently engaging in exercise, you can establish healthier habits and become a more productive individual, leading to a sense of fulfilment and well-being beyond your training sessions. This can lead to an overall improvement in your quality of life and contribute to a healthier and happier you. So not only does exercise have immediate benefits, but it can also have a positive impact on your future self.

Boxing can serve as a powerful outlet for emotional feelings, making it a valuable tool for personal growth and development. By channelling aggression into intense punch bag workouts, individuals can improve their punching power and technique while also managing their emotions in a healthy and positive way. In a sport where controlled aggression is necessary, boxing provides a safe and productive space for individuals to work through their feelings and improve themselves both physically and mentally. Whether it's releasing built-up stress or finding a healthy outlet for anger, boxing can be a beneficial outlet for emotional expression. It's important to find what works for you and utilize it in a positive manner, and boxing can be just that for many individuals.

While many people may view boxing as a physically aggressive sport, it can actually serve as a beneficial outlet for managing stress and anger. Engaging in a training routine and fully immersing yourself in the process can allow you to step away from any issues or challenges you may be facing and think through them rationally. Taking time for yourself, especially during times of heightened emotions, can be extremely helpful in managing your overall well-being. So, while boxing may involve physical strength and endurance, it can also be a powerful tool for mental and emotional health.

While boxing offers numerous benefits, it does not have to be a solitary activity. In fact, training in boxing often involves at least one other person. This can range from using focus pads with a trainer or sparring with an opponent to doing cardio exercises together for motivation and a more enjoyable experience. The camaraderie and support of a training partner can greatly enhance the overall experience and help push you to reach your goals. Additionally, having someone else to train with can also provide accountability and keep you on track with your fitness journey. So while boxing may be an individual sport, it doesn't mean you have to go it alone. Embrace the benefits of training with a partner and enjoy a more fulfilling and successful training experience.

Collaboration is key when it comes to training. Not only does working out with a partner enhance your physical performance and yield better results, but it also provides a space for open communication and the opportunity to make new friends. Having someone to train with allows you to share your thoughts and ideas while engaging in a productive training session. Whether it's discussing general life topics or specific ways to improve your training, the social aspect of training is a valuable experience. Don't hesitate to reach out and find a training partner to elevate your workouts and build a stronger support system.

The sport of boxing not only provides physical benefits, but it can also have a positive impact on mental health. Beyond the physical aspects, such as improved cardiovascular health and strength, boxing can help alleviate symptoms of anxiety and depression. Through the physical and mental challenges of training, individuals can gain a sense of accomplishment and increased confidence. Additionally, the supportive community and structure of a boxing gym can provide a sense of belonging and purpose, which can be especially beneficial for those struggling with mental health. Overall, boxing can be a valuable tool in managing and improving mental well-being.

In today's fast-paced world, finding time to focus on our physical well-being can be challenging. However, it's important to prioritize our health and fitness, and one way to do so is by finding a comfortable and safe space to exercise in our own ways and on our own time. Whether it's through a specific workout routine or simply taking some time out of our daily schedules to do something we enjoy, finding what works for us can greatly improve our self-confidence and esteem. Additionally, being able to train with friends or loved ones can add a social aspect to our fitness journey and make it even more enjoyable. So take the time to discover what works for you and make it a regular part of your routine. Your body and mind will thank you.

In addition to its numerous physical benefits, boxing also offers unique advantages that set it apart from other exercises. As you engage in boxing training, you will learn how to strategically plan and execute your workouts in order to reach your specific fitness goals. Whether you are aiming to increase strength while staying within weight classes, improve cardiovascular health, or lose weight, it is important to train smart and effectively. Boxing also allows you to develop and refine your technique, leading to the creation of your own individualized training and fighting style. Through this process, you will develop your own unique boxing persona and learn how to handle a variety of situations in order to maintain the upper hand. With boxing, you not only improve your physical health, but also develop valuable skills that can be applied to all aspects of your life.

26. Progressive muscle relaxation

Progressive muscle relaxation is a beneficial mind-body technique that involves the slow and deliberate tensing and relaxing of each muscle group in the body. Developed by physician Edmund Jacobson, it is often referred to as Jacobson's or deep muscle relaxation procedure. This technique is particularly useful in managing stress as it helps individuals become more aware of the physical sensations associated with tension. This heightened awareness allows for better recognition and management of everyday stress. Numerous studies have also shown that regular practice of progressive muscle relaxation can have positive effects on stress-related health issues, such as insomnia and anxiety. It is a simple yet effective tool for promoting overall well-being and managing the impact of stress on our bodies.

For an effective and beneficial progressive muscle relaxation session, it is important to find a comfortable position and a quiet space free of distractions. This allows you to fully focus on the exercise and reap its benefits. Start by tightening the muscles in your face for five seconds, including your eyes, forehead, and jaw. Then, take a deep breath and release the tension as you relax your face. Continue this process for the rest of your body, going through each muscle group one at a time. If you still feel tension in any muscles at the end, repeat the sequence at least three more times. By following these steps, you can experience the full effects of progressive muscle relaxation and achieve a state of relaxation and calm.

Several studies show that progressive muscle relaxation may help lessen stress. In a 2000 study from the Journal of Behavioural Medicine, for example, researchers exposed 67 volunteers to a stressful situation and then had them practice progressive muscle relaxation, undergo music therapy, or take part in a control group. Results revealed that members of the progressive muscle relaxation group experienced greater relaxation (including a more significant decrease in heart rate) than the rest of the study members. Other research indicates that progressive muscle relaxation may also help soothe stress by reducing levels of cortisol (a hormone released in response to stress).2 □

In addition, a number of studies suggest that progressive muscle relaxation may benefit people with certain health problems. For instance, a 2003 study from the journal Psych oncology found that progressive muscle relaxation helped relieve anxiety and improve quality of life among 29 colorectal cancer patients who had recently received surgery. A 2006 study published in the Journal of Alternative and Complementary Medicine, meanwhile, showed that progressive muscle relaxation improved quality of life and reduced blood pressure among people with heart disease.

27. Play

As adults, we often get caught up in the hustle and bustle of daily life and neglect to make time for pure enjoyment. Our focus is usually on work and family commitments, leaving little room for play. However, as we transition from childhood to adulthood, we tend to let go of the playful activities that brought us joy and rejuvenation. Instead, we opt for mindless activities like scrolling through social media or binge-watching TV shows. But play is not just reserved for children; it is a vital source of relaxation and stimulation for adults as well. Taking time to engage in fun and light-hearted activities can bring a much-needed break from the stress and responsibilities of adulthood. So don't forget to make time for play in your busy schedule, as it is essential for maintaining a healthy and balanced life.

Playing isn't just for kids – it's a crucial activity for adults as well. Whether it's with your romantic partner, friends, co-workers, pets, or children, engaging in playtime can have numerous benefits for your overall well-being. Not only does it help fuel your imagination and creativity, but it also enhances your problem-solving abilities and emotional health. When we engage in play, we can forget about our work and responsibilities and simply enjoy being social in an unstructured and creative way. So don't be afraid to set aside some time to play, as it can have a positive impact on all aspects of your life.

Taking time to play and let loose isn't just for kids anymore. As adults, we often get caught up in the responsibilities and stresses of everyday life, but it's important to make time for play. Whether it's goofing off with friends, playing with our pets, or simply enjoying a bike ride with no destination in mind, playing can bring joy and health benefits to our lives. It allows us to let go of our worries and stresses, and just be in the moment. So next time you have the urge to play, go ahead and embrace it with the same abandon and carefree attitude you had as a child. Your mind and body will thank you.

Play is often seen as an activity for children, but its benefits extend far beyond childhood. In fact, play can bring joy to our lives, reduce stress, enhance learning, and help us connect with others and the world around us. And it's not just for personal enjoyment - play can also improve productivity and satisfaction in our work. Whether it's a game of tag with friends or a creative project, incorporating play into our lives is essential for overall well-being and growth, no matter our age. So next time you feel guilty for taking a break to play, remember that it's actually benefiting your mental, emotional, and even professional well-being.

Playing is an essential part of life, and while it's great to play alone or with a furry companion, the benefits are even greater when playing with others. When we play with others, we engage in social interaction, communication, and teamwork. These skills are important for our overall well-being and development, and they can only be fully utilized when playing with others. Additionally, playing with others allows us to unplug from the constant sensory overload of electronic gadgets and truly connect with those around us. So, whether it's a game of catch, a board game, or a friendly competition, make sure to prioritize playtime with others for maximum benefits.

Integrating fun and play into your daily routine has proven to have a positive impact on various aspects of life, including relationships, mood, and overall outlook. In the midst of challenging times, taking a break from our troubles to engage in playful activities or share a laugh with others can significantly improve our well-being. As the saying goes, laughter truly is the best medicine. Not only does it bring joy and happiness in the moment, but its effects can also be long-lasting. By incorporating play and laughter into our lives, we can maintain a positive and optimistic mindset even during difficult situations, setbacks, or times of loss. It serves as a powerful tool in helping us cope and persevere through tough times.

It's never too late to tap into your playful and humorous side, even as an adult. Many of us tend to limit our playfulness out of fear of how we will be perceived by others. The concern of rejection, embarrassment, or ridicule is a valid one, but it shouldn't hold us back from expressing our light-heartedness. It's common for adults to worry that being playful will make them appear childish, but what's so wrong with that? Children possess an incredible amount of creativity, inventiveness, and a thirst for learning. Who wouldn't want to embrace those qualities? As children, we didn't worry about the opinions of others when we were playful. We can tap into that carefree nature again by setting aside time for quality play. The more we engage in play, jokes, and laughter, the easier it becomes to let go of our inhibitions and embrace our inner child.

In today's fast-paced world, it's important to take time for ourselves and unplug from the constant stimulation of technology. By clearing our schedules and turning off our devices, we give ourselves the opportunity to be fully present and indulge in activities that bring us joy. Give yourself the freedom to be spontaneous and let go of any inhibitions as you try something new and fun. Take a trip down memory lane and engage in an activity you haven't done since childhood. Embrace the change of pace and allow yourself to simply enjoy the present moment. It's a simple yet powerful way to recharge and refresh your mind and body. So go ahead and give yourself the gift of unplugging and embracing a little spontaneity. You deserve it.

28. Sex

The connection between sex and stress is a well-known fact that many of us have experienced first-hand. It's no surprise that high levels of stress can significantly decrease our sex drive, leaving us feeling uninterested and drained. However, it's also important to note that sex can be a great stress reliever. Despite the jokes about needing a good roll in the hay to cope with a difficult boss, there is some truth to it. Engaging in sexual activity can release endorphins and oxytocin, which can help reduce stress and promote relaxation. So, while stress may have a negative impact on our libido, it can also be used as a tool for stress relief and improving overall well-being.

The relationship between stress and sex has long been a topic of interest, and recent research has shed light on this intriguing connection. Studies have shown that a satisfying sex life can act as a natural stress reliever, reducing anxiety and tension. This may be due to the release of oxytocin, known as the love hormone, during sexual activity. Additionally, engaging in sexual activity can help improve sleep, boost mood, and increase overall feelings of well-being. However, it's important to note that the benefits of sex on stress relief are not one-size-fits-all and can vary from person to person. It's important to communicate openly and honestly with your partner and find what works best for you both in terms of stress management. With this in mind, incorporating a healthy and fulfilling sex life into your self-care routine may just be the perfect stress salve you've been looking for.

According to a study conducted by Arizona State University, engaging in physical affection or sexual behaviour with a partner can have a significant impact on a person's mood and stress levels. The study, which focused on 58 middle-aged women, found that these activities were associated with lower negative mood and stress levels and higher positive mood the following day. These findings suggest that physical intimacy with a partner can have positive effects on overall well-being and mental health. It's important to prioritize and maintain healthy relationships in order to experience these benefits.

In a recent study, researchers discovered a significant correlation between sex and decreased stress levels in women. Physical intimacy with a partner was found to lead to improved mood the following day. Interestingly, these results were not found when women experienced orgasms without a partner. This highlights the importance of the connection and emotional aspect of sex, rather than just the physical act itself. This study sheds light on the potential benefits of a healthy and fulfilling sexual relationship for women's overall well-being.

The results of a recent study have revealed a significant link between stress management and sexual activity. Not only does engaging in sexual activity lead to decreased levels of stress, but it also has a positive impact on one's overall mood. The study found that individuals in a good mood were more likely to engage in physical affection and sexual activity with their partner the following day. This highlights the cyclical nature of the sex-stress management connection, as sex can lead to decreased stress levels and decreased stress levels can lead to more sexual activity. These findings further emphasize the importance of effective stress management in maintaining a healthy and fulfilling sex life.

In another study, researchers looked at the impact of sexual intercourse on stress responses. Participants were exposed to two common stressors: public speaking and challenging math problems. The results showed that those who had recently engaged in sexual intercourse had lower baseline blood pressures and a smaller increase in blood pressure during the stressful tasks compared to those who had not recently engaged in sexual activity. This suggests that sexual intercourse may have a positive effect on managing stress and reducing the physiological response to stressors.

In a study analysing the stress responses of individuals during public speaking or challenging math problems, researchers found that those who had recently engaged in sexual intercourse showed lower baseline blood pressure levels and a decrease in blood pressure during stressful situations. This indicates that sexual activity may have a calming effect on the body, potentially reducing the physiological responses to stress. These findings further support the idea that sexual activity can have a positive impact on overall health and well-being.

A recent study delved into the effects of physical touch on women's stress levels and found that positive physical contact with a partner can significantly decrease stress response. This was measured through changes in heart rate and cortisol levels. Interestingly, emotional support alone did not have the same effect, emphasizing the importance of physical touch in providing comfort and reducing stress. These findings highlight the powerful impact of physical contact in promoting overall well-being and supporting individuals during times of stress.

Aside from the obvious pleasure it brings, orgasm also has numerous benefits for our health and stress relief. The release of hormones during orgasm can actually relax our bodies and contribute to overall wellness. In addition to the physical benefits, the emotional effects of orgasm can also be incredibly beneficial. It can provide a sense of relaxation and help reduce stress and anxiety. So next time you're feeling stressed or overwhelmed, don't overlook the power of orgasm to bring both physical and emotional relief.

Beyond its physical and emotional benefits, engaging in sexual activity can also have positive effects on stress management. Studies have shown that having sex can effectively take your mind off of worries for a significant period of time, allowing for a break from stressors. It also has the potential to release endorphins and promote relaxation, which can help reduce feelings of anxiety and tension. Furthermore, the emotional and physical connection with a partner during sex can help foster a sense of intimacy and closeness, which can have a positive impact on overall well-being. Overall, sex has clear stress management components that make it a beneficial activity for both physical and mental health.

One effective way to reduce stress and tension is through deep, relaxed breathing exercises. While these can certainly be done on your own, combining them with the pleasure and intimacy of sex with a loving partner can provide even greater benefits. Not only can this help manage stress, but it also adds a layer of enjoyment and connection to the experience. So why not incorporate both into your routine for a truly enjoyable and stress-relieving experience?

Numerous studies have shown that massage has a multitude of benefits, including being a great stress reliever. This is because humans need touch for our emotional health; in fact, studies have shown that babies who are not touched enough can fail to thrive. This need for touch continues into adulthood, making the type of relaxing, loving touch shared between partners an important way to reduce stress. Whether it's through a professional massage or a simple exchange of affection with a loved one, touch can have a powerful impact on our emotional well-being and stress levels.

The release of endorphins and other feel-good hormones during sexual activity can have a profound impact on both the body and mind. Not only can these chemicals create a sense of relaxation, but they can also leave us feeling better for hours afterward. It's truly remarkable how many hormones are involved in sexual activity and the various effects they have on our well-being. By understanding the science behind these feel-good chemicals, we can fully appreciate the benefits of engaging in sexual activity and the positive impact it can have on our overall health and happiness. So go ahead and indulge in some consensual and safe sexual activity, and reap the benefits of those feel-good hormones.

It's a common experience for individuals to notice a decrease in their sex drive when they're feeling stressed. However, there are ways to overcome this and get in the mood for sex with some intentional effort. It's important to remember that stress can take a toll on both our physical and mental well-being, so it's essential to address it and find ways to manage it. Some helpful tips include setting aside time for relaxation and self-care, communicating openly with your partner about your needs and boundaries, and finding ways to reduce stress in your daily life. With some conscious effort, it is possible to prioritize your sexual well-being and enjoy a fulfilling sex life, even during stressful times.

29. Walking

In addition to the physical benefits, walking and exercise can have positive impacts on mental and spiritual well-being. While many people engage in these activities to improve their physical health, the benefits extend far beyond just the physical realm. Taking a walk can help clear the mind and reduce stress and anxiety. It can also be a form of meditation, allowing for a sense of calm and inner peace. Exercise can also boost mood and self-esteem, leading to a more positive outlook on life. Whether you're walking for fitness or for mental and spiritual well-being, the benefits are undeniable. So don't underestimate the power of a good walk – it can do wonders for both the body and the mind.

There is growing evidence that walking can have numerous positive effects on both our physical and mental well-being. Studies have shown that walking can boost our mood, help us cope with life stress, and even work through relationship problems. Furthermore, many individuals have reported that walking has led to a deeper spiritual and religious life, providing a sense of calm and inner peace. So whether it's a brisk walk in the park or a leisurely stroll through your neighbourhood, incorporating walking into your daily routine can have a multitude of benefits for your overall health and well-being.

In our busy and hectic lives, stress is a common and often unavoidable experience. However, incorporating regular walks into your routine can greatly help to relieve stress. Not only does walking give you the physical activity your body needs, but it also provides a mental break from stressors. It allows you to step away from the environment that may be causing stress and gives you time to think and clear your mind. Breathing in fresh air and feeling your body move are natural stress-relievers, making walking an effective way to manage stress. So, the next time you feel overwhelmed, take a break and go for a walk. Your mind and body will thank you.

Other ways walking can relieve stress:

1. Take a Break: When it comes to managing stress, one effective strategy is to physically and mentally distance yourself from the stressful environment. This can involve getting up and taking a 15-

minute walking break, whether it's around the office or outside in nature. This simple action can help clear your mind and provide a much-needed break from the stressors that are causing you anxiety. By physically moving away from the source of stress, you are also creating mental distance, giving yourself a chance to refocus and approach the situation with a calmer mindset. So the next time you're feeling overwhelmed, don't be afraid to take a walk and give yourself some distance to decompress and recharge.

2. Loosen Up: As many of us know, stress can manifest itself in our bodies by causing tension in our muscles. However, one effective way to alleviate this tension is by focusing on proper walking posture and form. By consciously engaging our muscles in this way, we can actually release the knots and put them to work in a beneficial manner. For even greater relaxation in the shoulders and neck, consider incorporating the Nordic walking technique with fitness walking poles. Not only will this provide a physical release of tension, but it can also improve our overall well-being and reduce stress levels. Give it a try and see the difference it can make in your daily life.

3. Get Out of Your Head: In the midst of our busy and often stressful lives, it's important to take a break from our internal worries and focus on the world around us. Take a moment to observe the environment around you and appreciate the natural beauty that surrounds us. Take a walk and enjoy the trees, flowers, and birds, or simply sit and take in the view of a garden or the sky. Even window shopping can provide a welcome distraction as you stroll past storefronts or explore a shopping centre. These simple actions can help to clear our minds and bring a sense of calm and peace to our day. So the next time you feel overwhelmed, take a moment to pause and enjoy the world around you.

4. Reconnect With Your Physical Body: It's important to take a holistic approach to our bodies, from head to toe. Our bodies are constantly working to carry us along, and we can support them by practicing breathing techniques and improving our walking form. And while we do this, let's take a moment to truly appreciate our surroundings. Feel the warmth of the sun, the gentle breeze, the refreshing mist, or the invigorating rain on your skin. This mindful appreciation of our body and environment can lead to a deeper connection with ourselves and the world around us.

5. Burn Calories From Stress-Eating: During times of stress, it's not uncommon to turn to unhealthy comfort foods or convenient, high-calorie options. However, a simple solution to combat these habits is to get up and get moving. Walking is a great way to burn calories without having to change into workout gear or hit the gym. It's a low-impact exercise that can be done almost anywhere and can help improve overall physical and mental health. So next time you're feeling overwhelmed or tempted to indulge in unhealthy foods, take a walk instead. Your body and mind will thank you.

6. Time to Think: "All truly great thoughts are conceived while walking," said philosopher Friedrich Nietzsche. One of the most beneficial activities you can do for your brain is to simply take a walk. This allows for an increase in blood flow to your brain, giving you the mental space and clarity to consider different aspects of your problems without the distractions of your office or home. As you walk, you may find that creative ideas and solutions flow more easily, allowing you to come up with innovative solutions to your challenges. By taking the time to disconnect from your daily surroundings and engage in physical activity, you are giving your brain the opportunity to rejuvenate and problem-solve in a more effective and efficient manner. So next time you feel stuck, try taking a walk and see how it can positively impact your thinking process.

7. Talk and Laugh: Stress can often consume our thoughts and affect our mood, making it difficult to fully enjoy the simple things in life. That's why choosing a fun walking companion can be so beneficial. Not only will they provide a welcome distraction from the things causing you stress, but they can also bring out your happy side. Let them entertain you with their playful antics and make you forget your worries for a while. As you walk, take advantage of any playgrounds you might pass by and be silly with your companion. Laugh, run, and have fun together. You'll be surprised at how much lighter you'll feel after a fun and carefree walk with a furry friend by your side.

8. Vent: When looking for a walking companion to help you manage stress, it's important to choose someone who is willing to listen and provide emotional support and advice. Seek out a person who is skilled in problem-solving and counselling, as this can lead to more productive and effective conversations. A good walking companion will not only listen to what is causing your stress, but also offer helpful insights and guidance on how to manage and overcome it. Having a supportive and understanding companion by your side during walks can make a significant difference in your overall well-being and stress management. So choose wisely and find a companion who can truly be a source of comfort and assistance on your journey to better mental health.

9. Widen Your Vision: It's no secret that stress can be all-consuming, causing us to only focus on our immediate problems and concerns. However, taking a step back and observing our surroundings can help broaden our perspective and remind us that there is more to life than just our own issues. Whether it's taking a walk around the neighbourhood or simply looking out the window, paying attention to what is going on around us can help us see that there is a world outside of our own problems. We may notice new neighbours moving in, co-workers preparing for a party, or even a new walking path being built. These observations can help us realize that there is more going on in the world and remind us to take a break from our stress and enjoy the present moment.

10. Lower Your Blood Pressure: The connection between stress and high blood pressure is well-documented, and managing stress levels is crucial for maintaining overall health. Fortunately, studies have shown that something as simple as walking can have a positive impact on both blood pressure and heart health. In fact, research has found that incorporating a daily walking routine can significantly lower blood pressure and reduce the risk of heart disease. So next time you're feeling stressed, take a walk and prioritize your physical and mental well-being. Your body will thank you.

11. Walk in a Park for Increased Stress Relief: According to recent studies, spending time in a natural environment can have a significantly positive impact on stress levels. In fact, research has shown that walking in a natural environment can have a greater effect on stress relief than walking in an urban setting. This highlights the importance of incorporating nature into our daily lives, whether it's taking a walk in a park or simply spending some time in a garden. These findings have significant implications for mental health and overall well-being, emphasizing the need for individuals to have access to natural environments in their daily routines.

Regular exercise, including walking, has been proven to have a positive impact on our mood. This is because physical activity triggers the release of endorphins, also known as the body's natural happy drugs. People who walk at a brisk pace and raise their heart rate will likely experience this effect even more strongly. However, even those who walk at a slower pace will still notice an improvement in their mood. So, whether you prefer a brisk walk or a leisurely stroll, incorporating walking into your routine can have a significant impact on your overall well-being.

According to numerous physicians, incorporating regular walking and exercise into your daily routine can be a beneficial natural treatment for relieving symptoms of depression. This is because depression is often linked to brain chemistry, and physical activity can trigger the release of endorphins, the happy chemicals that prescription drugs and herbs aim to stimulate artificially. By engaging in regular exercise, you can naturally achieve the same positive effects on your mood without relying on medication. So, next time you're feeling down, try going for a walk or getting some exercise to boost your endorphin levels and lift your spirits.

It's important to recognize that depression is a serious illness that can have severe consequences, which is why it's crucial to consult a health care provider if you are experiencing symptoms. These may include changes in mood, behaviour, and thoughts, as well as feelings of hopelessness and worthlessness. If left untreated, depression can lead to serious problems in one's life, and in extreme cases, suicidal thoughts. As a part of effective treatment for mood disorders, incorporating physical activity, such as walking, can be beneficial. This can be used in conjunction with other treatment methods, such as talk therapy and medication, to improve overall well-being and manage symptoms of depression. If you or a loved one are struggling with depression, seek professional help and explore different treatment options to find what works best for you. Regular exercise, particularly walking, has been proven to have significant benefits for the brain. In fact, a study conducted in 1999 on individuals over the age of 60 showed that walking for 45 minutes a day at a 16-minute mile pace led to improvements in cognitive abilities. The participants in the study gradually increased their walking time and speed, starting at just 15 minutes of walking. The results were remarkable, with the participants experiencing a boost in mental sharpness after incorporating this walking program into their daily routine. So, not only does walking improve physical health, but it also has positive effects on brain function.

The benefits of exercise on our physical health are well-known, but it turns out it's just as important for our mental health as well. According to a study conducted in 2011, older adults who walked for 40 minutes a day, three times a week, not only reduced the normal age-related shrinkage of the brain's hippocampus (where memory and emotions are processed), but also improved their performance on spatial memory tasks after a year. This goes to show that incorporating regular physical activity into our routines can have significant impacts on our brain health and overall cognitive function, making it a crucial aspect of healthy aging. So let's lace up our trainers and take a walk for the sake of our minds and bodies.

30. Breathing exercises

Incorporating breathing exercises into your daily routine can greatly improve your overall sense of relaxation. Take a moment to notice how your body feels when you are in a state of relaxation, whether it be first thing in the morning or just before you fall asleep. You may notice a slow and steady breath, a sense of calm, and a release of tension in your muscles. By focusing on your breathing, you can replicate this feeling of relaxation whenever you need it. Breathing exercises can be especially helpful during times of stress, as they can help you to feel more centred and calmer. So the next time you are feeling overwhelmed, take a few moments to focus on your breath and allow your body to relax.

Taking a moment to focus on your breath can have powerful effects on reducing stress and tension in the body. Deep breathing sends a signal to the brain to relax, which in turn calms the body and decreases heart rate, breathing rate, and blood pressure. It's no wonder that breathing exercises are often recommended as a way to manage stress. The beauty of these exercises is that they are easy to learn and can be done anytime, anywhere without any special equipment. By trying out different exercises, you can find the ones that work best for you and make them a part of your regular routine for stress relief. Remember, the way you breathe can have a profound impact on your overall well-being. So take a deep breath and let go of your stress and tension.

There are lots of breathing exercises you can do to help relax. The first exercise below—belly breathing—is simple to learn and easy to do. It's best to start there if you have never done breathing exercises before. The other exercises are more advanced. All of these exercises can help you relax and relieve stress.

Belly breathing

Belly breathing is easy to do and very relaxing. Try this basic exercise anytime you need to relax or relieve stress.
Sit or lie flat in a comfortable position.

Put one hand on your belly just below your ribs and the other hand on your chest.
Take a deep breath in through your nose, and let your belly push your hand out. Your chest should not move.
Breathe out through pursed lips as if you were whistling. Feel the hand on your belly go in and use it to push all the air out.
Do this breathing 3 to 10 times. Take your time with each breath.
Notice how you feel at the end of the exercise.

Next steps

After you have mastered belly breathing, you may want to try one of these more advanced breathing exercises. Try all three, and see which one works best for you:
4-7-8 breathing
Roll breathing
Morning breathing
4-7-8 breathing
This exercise also uses belly breathing to help you relax. You can do this exercise either sitting or lying down.
To start, put one hand on your belly and the other on your chest as in the belly breathing exercise.
Take a deep, slow breath from your belly, and silently count to 4 as you breathe in.
Hold your breath, and silently count from 1 to 7.
Breathe out completely as you silently count from 1 to 8. Try to get all the air out of your lungs by the time you count to 8.
Repeat 3 to 7 times or until you feel calm.
Notice how you feel at the end of the exercise.

Roll breathing

Roll breathing helps you to develop full use of your lungs and to focus on the rhythm of your breathing. You can do it in any position. But while you are learning, it is best to lie on your back with your knees bent.
Put your left hand on your belly and your right hand on your chest. Notice how your hands move as you breathe in and out.

Practice filling your lower lungs by breathing so that your "belly" (left) hand goes up when you inhale and your "chest" (right) hand remains still. Always breathe in through your nose and breathe out through your mouth. Do this 8 to 10 times.

When you have filled and emptied your lower lungs 8 to 10 times, add the second step to your breathing: inhale first into your lower lungs as before, and then continue inhaling into your upper chest. Breathe slowly and regularly. As you do so, your right hand will rise, and your left hand will fall a little as your belly falls.

As you exhale slowly through your mouth, make a quiet, whooshing sound as first your left hand and then your right-hand fall. As you exhale, feel the tension leaving your body as you become more and more relaxed.

Practice breathing in and out in this way for 3 to 5 minutes. Notice that the movement of your belly and chest rises and falls like the motion of rolling waves.

Notice how you feel at the end of the exercise.

Practice roll breathing daily for several weeks until you can do it almost anywhere. You can use it as an instant relaxation tool anytime you need one.

Caution: Some people get dizzy the first few times they try roll breathing. If you begin to breathe too fast or feel lightheaded, slow your breathing. Get up slowly.

Morning breathing

Try this exercise when you first get up in the morning to relieve muscle stiffness and clear clogged breathing passages. Then use it throughout the day to relieve back tension.

From a standing position, bend forward from the waist with your knees slightly bent, letting your arms dangle close to the floor.

As you inhale slowly and deeply, return to a standing position by rolling up slowing, lifting your head last.

Hold your breath for just a few seconds in this standing position.

Exhale slowly as you return to the original position, bending forward from the waist.

Notice how you feel at the end of the exercise.

31. Take a Sauna

In recent years, the popularity of saunas has grown significantly, and this trend is seen worldwide. While many may wonder where this practice originated from, it is primarily attributed to Europe and the Nordic region. In fact, Finnish sauna culture is well-established and widely recognized. Saunas are traditionally small houses or rooms that are specifically designed for heat sessions, which can be either dry or wet. Regular sauna sessions have been linked to numerous health benefits, which explains the growing demand for this form of relaxation.

What are the health benefits of the sauna?

Regular use of a sauna has numerous benefits, one of which is boosting the immune system. This is because saunas induce a mild fever, which activates the body's immune response and increases the production of white blood cells. Additionally, the heat and steam from the sauna can help clear the sinuses and respiratory passages, preventing illnesses such as colds and flu. The relaxation and stress-reducing effects of sauna use also contribute to a stronger immune system, as stress can weaken the body's ability to fight off infections. Overall, incorporating sauna sessions into your routine can help improve your overall health and wellness by strengthening your immune system.

Using a sauna on a regular basis has been proven to have numerous health benefits, one of which is boosting the body's production of white blood cells. These cells play a crucial role in fighting off infections and illnesses. Studies have shown that individuals who use a sauna frequently have a higher count of white blood cells, leading to a stronger immune system and a better ability to combat infections. By regularly using a sauna, individuals can maintain their health and prevent illness by strengthening their body's natural defence system. This is just one of the many positive effects that sauna use can have on the body.

Using a sauna can have numerous benefits for both the body and mind. One of the most significant advantages is its ability to help us adapt to stress and decrease the risk of mental health disorders like depression. By creating a warm and peaceful environment free from external distractions, saunas offer a form of stress relief that can be incredibly beneficial. This quiet and calming space allows for a much-needed break from the outside world, promoting relaxation and aiding in the reduction of stress levels. Overall, incorporating sauna use into your routine can have a positive impact on your overall well-being.

One of the most beneficial aspects of using a sauna is its ability to relax the body's muscles. The heat from the sauna penetrates deep into the muscles, relieving tension and promoting a sense of calm. Additionally, sauna use has been shown to improve circulation, helping to oxygenate the body and provide a natural detox. But perhaps one of the best-known benefits of sauna use is the release of endorphins, our body's feel-good chemical. This release creates a sense of euphoria and relaxation, often referred to as the after-sauna glow. With these amazing benefits, it's no wonder saunas have been used for centuries for their therapeutic effects.

For those of us who do not regularly engage in physical activity, deep sweating may seem like an unattainable goal. However, regular sauna bathing is a great way to reap the numerous health benefits of deep sweating. As the heat of a sauna raises our core body temperature, we begin to sweat, allowing our bodies to eliminate toxins and detoxify. This can have a positive impact on our overall health and well-being. So if you're looking for a way to incorporate deep sweating into your routine, consider adding regular sauna sessions to your schedule. Your body will thank you for it.

For centuries, heat bathing has been utilized as a beauty and health strategy for maintaining healthy skin. The process of deep sweating helps to cleanse the skin by removing dead skin cells and replacing them with new ones. As the body sweats, bacteria is flushed out of the pores and sweat ducts, promoting a healthier epidermal layer. The act of cleansing the pores through heat bathing has also been proven to improve capillary circulation, resulting in a softer and more radiant complexion. This age-old technique is a natural and effective way to keep your skin in good condition and maintain its youthful appearance.

Studies have demonstrated that sauna use can lead to a more restful and rejuvenating sleep. The release of endorphins, along with the increase in body temperature during sauna sessions, creates a gradual and relaxing decline in endorphins, which is crucial in promoting quality sleep. Many sauna users from all over the world have reported experiencing a deep and restful sleep after taking a sauna bath, thanks to the calming and soothing effects of the heat. So, if you're looking to improve your sleep, incorporating sauna sessions into your routine may be worth considering.

32. Aromatherapy

The rise of aromatherapy in recent years has been quite remarkable. From once being seen as an exotic practice, it is now a mainstream industry with products available even in grocery stores. Aromatherapy candles, bath products, essential oils, and other items are now easily accessible and are said to have various benefits such as soothing babies, relieving stress, and promoting healthy living. But as with any trend, the question remains: does aromatherapy truly live up to its claims? While the use of scents for therapeutic purposes is not a new concept, it is important to carefully evaluate the effectiveness and safety of these products before incorporating them into our daily routines. With the growing popularity of aromatherapy, it is crucial to gather reliable information and make informed decisions about its use.

Despite the limited amount of research available on aromatherapy, there have been significant findings that support its effectiveness in relieving stress. Studies have shown that aromatherapy can alter brain waves and behaviour, reduce the perception of stress, and decrease levels of the stress hormone cortisol. Additionally, lavender aromatherapy has been proven to reduce crying in infants and promote sleep in both infants and adults. Different scents can also have varying effects on individuals, and one study even found that aromatherapy massage can provide relief from anxiety and depression. Furthermore, combining massage with aromatherapy has been shown to provide stronger and more continuous relief from mental fatigue compared to massage alone. While further research is needed, these findings suggest that aromatherapy can be a beneficial tool in managing stress.

In the realm of stress relief, aromatherapy may not be a magic cure, but it has been shown to have positive effects. This makes it a great tool to have in your stress relief arsenal. Not only does aromatherapy have few known side effects, but it can also be used passively. This means that you can simply fill the room with a soothing scent while you go about your day, allowing it to work its stress-relieving magic in the background. Furthermore, aromatherapy can easily be combined with other stress-relieving techniques, such as massage or meditation, for even greater benefits. With a wide range of aromatherapy products available, it's a convenient option for anyone looking to incorporate stress relief into their daily routine.

Aromatherapy can be convenient, especially for busy people who need something quick. Here are some ideas for aromatherapy use:
Candles have become increasingly popular for their benefits in aromatherapy. By simply lighting a candle, you can easily infuse a room with a pleasant scent and create a calming ambiance. Aromatherapy candles are a great option for those looking to enhance their meditation practice or create a more relaxing environment. Unlike incense, candles produce less smoke and can be more practical for everyday use. So next time you want to create a soothing atmosphere, consider lighting an aromatherapy candle for a subtle yet effective method.

Be sure that you get quality candles that give off a scent that's potent enough to be smelled around the room.
Aromatherapy diffusers are a popular method of using essential oils to create a soothing atmosphere. These diffusers work by evaporating the oils into the air, using either a candle or batteries. This allows the scent to spread effectively and create a calming environment. Many people prefer battery-operated diffusers for their safety, as there is no open flame involved. Additionally, diffusers can add to the overall aesthetic of a room, enhancing the soothing vibe they are intended to create. Whether you opt for a diffuser with a candle or battery-powered, it is a convenient and effective way to enjoy the benefits of aromatherapy.
One of the best things about aromatherapy body products is their ability to create a personal scent that lingers on your skin without being overpowering to others. Whether you prefer a full-body application of aromatherapy lotion or a few drops of skin-safe essential oils on your pulse points, you can enjoy the scent for hours. This discreet and personal touch makes aromatherapy body products perfect for any occasion, whether it be a busy day at work or a night out with friends. So go ahead and indulge in the soothing scents of aromatherapy without worrying about bothering others.

Research has shown that combining aromatherapy with massage can have even greater benefits than using either strategy alone. If you have a willing partner, trading aromatherapy massages can be a cost-effective and enjoyable way to reduce stress. However, if this is not an option, investing in a professional massage can be well worth the money. By incorporating aromatherapy into a massage, you can enhance the relaxation and therapeutic effects, leading to a more satisfying and rejuvenating experience. So why not give it a try and reap the benefits of this powerful stress-relieving combination?

Incorporating aromatherapy into your meditation practice can have numerous benefits for both your mind and body. The use of scents, such as incense or essential oils, can enhance the relaxation experienced during meditation and provide a focal point for your thoughts. Additionally, the passive stress relief offered by aromatherapy can aid in achieving a deeper state of calm and clarity. It only takes five minutes to experience the benefits of meditation, so why not try the calming aromas of incense or a soothing bath to enhance your practice? Whether it's through the use of incense or essential oils, aromatherapy can be a valuable tool in achieving a more peaceful and centred state of mind.

33. Take a warm bath

In today's fast-paced and busy world, taking the time for a good bath may seem like a luxury. However, beyond just a form of essential self-care, studies have shown that it can actually have numerous benefits for your mental health. From reducing stress and anxiety to improving overall mood and even aiding in better sleep, a relaxing bath can do wonders for our well-being. In fact, research has shown that soaking in warm water can trigger the release of endorphins, which are natural feel-good chemicals in our brains. So next time you feel overwhelmed or just need a moment of peace, don't hesitate to treat yourself to a good, warm bath. It's not just a luxury, it's a scientifically proven way to improve your mental health.

From ancient civilizations to modern times, bathing has held a significant role in societies around the world. Beyond just maintaining personal hygiene, cleanliness has long been associated with power and beauty. In fact, public baths were not only a way to get clean, but also a means of socializing and building communities. Throughout history, bathing has been more than just a daily routine – it has been a cultural practice that brings people together. Even today, the act of taking a bath or shower is still viewed as a way to refresh and rejuvenate oneself, both physically and mentally. The significance of bathing goes far beyond just getting clean; it is a reflection of our societal values and norms.

The simple act of taking a hot bubble bath has evolved from a necessary means of cleanliness to a form of self-care and relaxation. In today's fast-paced world, many of us turn to a hot bath as a way to unwind after a long and stressful day or to soothe our muscles after a tough workout. However, recent studies have shown that the benefits of bathing go beyond just a temporary escape from reality. Not only does a hot bath improve skin health, but it also has a positive impact on our mental and emotional well-being. So next time you feel guilty for taking a long soak in the tub, remember that it's not just a luxury, but a beneficial practice for your overall health.

Recent research from Germany has revealed a surprising solution for depression - hot baths. In a study, participants who suffered from depression reported feeling a significant improvement in mood after soaking in a 40C bath for just 30 minutes. In fact, the results showed that regular baths were even more effective in treating depression than aerobic exercise. This new finding highlights the potential benefits of using hot baths as a non-invasive and enjoyable method for managing depression. Further research and exploration of this therapy could potentially provide a simple and accessible solution for those struggling with depression.

A study conducted in Japan delved into the potential mental health benefits of bathing compared to showering. The results showed that those who took a bath experienced reduced levels of stress, tension-anxiety, anger-hostility, and depression. This further supports the notion that taking a bath can have a positive impact on our mental well-being. Whether it's the warm water, soothing scents, or the act of relaxation, there seems to be a correlation between bathing and improved mental health. This information could be valuable for individuals looking for natural and accessible ways to manage their stress and improve their overall mood.

According to recent studies, taking a hot bath before bed can have significant benefits on our sleep and overall wellbeing. The warmth of the water helps to increase our body temperature, which in turn helps to regulate our circadian rhythms and improve the quality of our sleep. This can lead to a more restful night's sleep and an overall feeling of improved wellbeing. By taking a hot bath before bed, we are able to tap into the natural power of our body's internal clock and create a more harmonious balance between our sleep and waking patterns. So next time you're struggling to get a good night's rest, consider taking a relaxing and rejuvenating hot bath to help you wind down and prepare for a restful night's sleep.

Before you get lathered up, here are a few tips on how to create a soothing experience that will help you rebalance in the comfort of your own home.

As adults, it's important to take a bath that is between 40–45C for optimal health. This temperature range, paired with a room temperature of 25C, creates the perfect balance for increasing body temperature in a comfortable and controlled manner. By reducing cold stress from the exterior environment, this magical combination allows for a relaxing and beneficial bathing experience. Whether it's a warm soak after a long day or a soothing bath to destress, keeping the water and room temperatures within these ranges will ensure a healthy and enjoyable experience.

A good night's sleep is crucial for our overall well-being, and essential oils can help promote a restful slumber. Ylang ylang is known for its calming properties, making it a great choice for those struggling with sleep issues. For a more invigorating experience, citrus oils like petitgrain or bergamot can help uplift your mood and increase alertness. But why stop there? Adding fresh rose petals to your bathwater not only creates a beautiful aesthetic, but it also releases a soothing rosewater scent that is suitable for even the most sensitive skin. So why not enhance your relaxation routine with the power of essential oils and rose petals? Sweet dreams await.

When using essential oils, it is crucial to dilute them with a carrier oil to prevent any potential skin irritation. This is especially important when making a 2% dilution, which is a common ratio for topical application. A simple rule to follow is to add 12 drops of essential oil per 30ml of carrier oil. This will ensure a safe and effective application of the essential oil without any risk of adverse reactions. Always remember to take the necessary precautions when working with essential oils to ensure a positive and enjoyable experience.

In today's modern world, we are constantly surrounded by blue light from our electronic devices, leading to mental fatigue and headaches. However, there is a simple solution to combat this issue – taking a bath. For a refreshing daytime bath, try using your bathroom's natural light for a luxurious experience. Not only does this feel like a pampering treat, but exposure to natural light can also improve your overall sense of wellbeing and promote better sleep. For a relaxing evening bath, consider turning off the lights and bathing by candlelight. This can help regulate your body's production of melatonin, which is often suppressed by artificial light at night, leading to better sleep quality and timing. So the next time you're feeling overwhelmed by blue light, remember the simple but effective solution of taking a bath.

As tempting as it may be to catch up on your favourite Netflix shows while soaking in the tub with your iPad propped up, we highly recommend leaving technology out of the equation. The blue light emitted from screens can disrupt your body's natural rhythms and make it difficult to relax. Instead, embrace the peace and quiet or surround yourself with the soothing sounds of nature, such as rainforest noises or ocean waves. Studies have shown that these sounds can decrease the body's stress response and increase feelings of relaxation, making your bath time even more enjoyable and beneficial for your well-being. So next time you reach for your iPad, try embracing the calming effects of nature instead.

For those who have difficulty meditating in traditional settings, a relaxing bath may be the perfect alternative. The warm water and comfortable position of the body naturally induce a state of relaxation, making it easier to clear the mind and find peace in your own personal oasis. With your eyes closed, take slow and deep breaths, and focus on the present moment. Pay attention to the soothing sound of the water and the calming aroma of essential oils. Allow yourself to completely unwind and embrace a sense of complete relaxation.

34. Soothing music

For centuries, music has been known to have a profound impact on our emotions and well-being. In fact, the power of music to soothe and calm us is widely recognized and has been used as a stress management tool for many years. This unique link between music and our emotions has been extensively studied and the results consistently show its effectiveness in reducing stress levels. Whether it's through listening to our favourite songs or playing an instrument, incorporating music into our daily lives can greatly improve our overall mental and emotional health. Its ability to evoke specific emotions and create a sense of relaxation makes music a valuable tool for managing stress and promoting overall well-being.

As a stress management tool, listening to slow, quiet classical music can have a tremendous effect on both our minds and bodies. The soothing melodies and gentle rhythms have been found to slow our pulse and heart rate, lower blood pressure, and decrease the levels of stress hormones in our bodies. It's no wonder that music has been used for centuries as a way to relax and unwind. Whether you're looking to wind down after a long day or find a moment of calm amidst a busy schedule, music can be a powerful tool in helping you achieve a state of relaxation and tranquillity. So the next time you're feeling overwhelmed, turn on some slow, quiet classical music and let its peaceful melodies wash over you.

In today's fast-paced world, it can be challenging to find moments of peace and stillness. This is where music can come in as a powerful tool for meditation. Not only does it capture our attention, but it also helps us to delve deeper into our emotions and inner thoughts. With its soothing and rhythmic qualities, music can help prevent our minds from wandering during meditation, allowing us to stay present and focused. Whether it's instrumental music or calming vocals, incorporating music into your meditation practice can greatly enhance the experience and provide a deeper sense of relaxation. So the next time you're looking to meditate, consider turning on some calming tunes to help guide you towards a more mindful state.

As individuals, we all have our own unique preferences when it comes to music. What may be calming for one person may not have the same effect on another. This is why it's important to choose music that speaks to you and is suitable for your mood. While you may not typically listen to classical music, it may be worth giving it a try when seeking a sense of calmness. With its soothing melodies and peaceful rhythms, classical music has been known to have a calming effect on the mind and body. So, when in doubt, why not give it a chance and see if it helps to ease your mind and create a peaceful atmosphere.

In times of high stress, many individuals may find themselves avoiding music as a means of coping. They may view it as a frivolous activity that does not contribute to their productivity or overall well-being. However, research has shown that actively listening to music can actually reduce stress levels and increase productivity. By taking the time to incorporate music into your daily routine, even in small doses, you can reap the benefits of improved focus and reduced stress. So why not give it a try and see how it positively impacts your productivity and overall mindset? The rewards may be more significant than you think.

Incorporating music into our daily routines can have a positive impact on our overall well-being, especially for those dealing with clinical depression or bipolar disorder. One way to do this is by playing a playlist or the radio while in the car or taking portable music with you while walking the dog. Another option is to turn on music instead of the TV, whether it be during bath or shower time or just in the background while completing daily tasks. Music has the power to uplift our moods and provide a sense of comfort and distraction during difficult times, making it a helpful tool in managing mental health.

For many, singing along to their favourite songs can be a great way to release tension and let go of stress. It's also a fun and enjoyable activity for extroverts, making karaoke a popular pastime. Additionally, listening to calming music before bedtime can promote feelings of peace and relaxation, making it easier to fall asleep. This is especially helpful for those who struggle with winding down after a long day. So whether it's belting out your favourite tunes or winding down with soothing melodies, music can be a powerful tool for managing emotions and promoting overall well-being.

Research on Music

For centuries, music has been recognized for its healing properties and its ability to bring harmony between mind and body. While this has long been a belief, recent scientific studies have delved deeper into the potential benefits of music. These studies have found that music can bring a sense of order and security to disabled and distressed children, improving their coordination and communication skills and overall quality of life. Additionally, listening to music on headphones has been shown to reduce stress and anxiety in hospital patients both before and after surgery. It has also been found to alleviate both chronic and postoperative pain. Furthermore, music has been shown to have a positive impact on elderly individuals, reducing depression and increasing self-esteem. Even for nursing students, making music has been found to decrease burnout and improve mood. And for adult cancer patients, music therapy has been proven to significantly reduce emotional distress and enhance their quality of life. With all of these findings, it's clear that music has the power to heal and improve the lives of individuals of all ages and backgrounds.

Meditation

In the world of meditation, music can be a powerful tool to help slow down the mind and trigger the relaxation response. However, not all types of peaceful or New Age music will have the same effect on everyone. Music with no structure can be more distracting or even unsettling, while gentle music with a familiar melody tends to be more comforting. That being said, it's important to search for the type of music that personally produces a sense of calm, familiarity, and centeredness for each individual. With so many options available, it's worth taking the time to find the perfect soundtrack for your meditation practice.

Many individuals find that incorporating the sounds of nature into their daily lives can be a beneficial way to relax and unwind.

Whether it's the gentle trickling of water or the melodic chirping of birds, these natural sounds can help create a sense of calm and tranquillity. They can transport us to a peaceful setting, such as lying beside a mountain stream on a warm spring day, and aid in slowing down our busy minds and releasing stressful thoughts. Including nature's melodies in playlists specifically designed for relaxation is a popular practice and can be a useful tool in promoting a sense of peace   and   relaxation.

35. Take a Nap

As professionals, we are often conditioned to believe that being busy and working nonstop is the key to success. However, this mentality can lead to burnout and decreased productivity. Many of us experience a midday slump, where we feel tired and unproductive after lunch. This is a natural response to our circadian rhythm and can be remedied by taking a nap. In fact, research has shown that taking a short nap during the day can improve cognitive function, memory, and alertness. So instead of pushing through the fatigue, it may be time to listen to our bodies and take a much-needed break. Embracing rest and relaxation can ultimately lead to better productivity and overall well-being.

According to experts, taking a nap can have a multitude of benefits for our overall health. Not only does it boost our memory and increase creativity, but it also reduces stress. In fact, napping is a simple yet effective way to maintain our well-being. Instead of reaching for a cup of coffee or an energy drink, consider taking a quick nap to recharge and tackle the second half of the day with renewed energy. This habit can greatly improve our productivity and overall health in the long run. So next time you feel tired or overwhelmed, don't hesitate to take a short nap and reap the benefits.

According to Bill Anthony, an American psychologist and director of the Harvard University Psychiatric Rehabilitation Centre, napping can have numerous benefits as a form of stress relief. Having studied this topic for 20 years, Anthony asserts that napping not only improves our immune defences but also significantly reduces cortisol, the stress hormone. In addition, it has been shown to aid in memorization and brain renewal, making it easier to assimilate new information. Studies have also found that a 20-minute nap can boost creativity and increase intellectual capacities by up to 20 percent. This short amount of sleep can even have the same benefits as two hours of sleep when practiced daily. Clearly, incorporating a 20-minute nap into our daily routine can have a positive impact on our overall well-being.

Below are some secrets for a good nap:

Despite what many people may think, taking a nap is not just reserved for bedtime. In fact, naps can be taken in a variety of places such as a comfortable chair, a relaxing hammock, or even a cosy sofa. The key is to find a quiet and peaceful environment to help you unwind and recharge. By isolating yourself from noise, you can truly relax and reap the benefits of a refreshing nap. So don't feel guilty for taking a nap outside of your bed, find a comfortable spot and enjoy a moment of relaxation. Your mind and body will thank you for it.

Creating a peaceful and uninterrupted environment is key to falling asleep quickly. To eliminate any fear of being disturbed, it's important to turn off your phone and possibly close and lock the door of the room where you will be resting. By doing this, you can ensure that you won't be disturbed for about 20 minutes, allowing your mind to relax and your body to drift off into a peaceful sleep. This small adjustment can make a big difference in your ability to fall asleep quickly and wake up feeling refreshed. So take the time to set up a quiet and undisturbed space for yourself before bed, and watch as your sleep quality improves.

In order to wake up feeling well-rested and rejuvenated, it's important to avoid sending conflicting signals to your body. This means not plunging yourself into complete darkness, but rather leaving your blinds open and using a sleep mask if the light is bothersome. By keeping the blinds open, you are allowing your body to naturally adjust to the rising sun, signalling to your brain that it's time to wake up. Using a sleep mask can help block out any excess light and ensure that you get the quality sleep your body needs. Remember, consistency is key when it comes to a good night's rest, so make sure to keep your blinds open and use a sleep mask if needed to maintain a healthy sleep schedule.

As we all know, getting a good night's sleep is essential for our overall health and well-being. And in order to achieve that, our body needs to be as relaxed as possible. So before hitting the sheets, make sure to take a moment to loosen up. This could mean undoing your tie or unbuttoning your shirt to allow for better circulation and comfort. It's also important to avoid crossing your legs, as this can restrict blood flow and lead to discomfort or even cramping. By following these simple steps, you can ensure that your body is in the most relaxed state possible, allowing you to dive into a peaceful slumber and wake up feeling refreshed and rejuvenated.

As individuals, we all have different sleep schedules and it's important to listen to our own biological clock when deciding on the perfect time to take a nap. Many people experience drowsiness after lunch, around 2:00 to 3:00, making it an ideal time for a nap. However, it's important to avoid napping after 5 p.m. as this can interfere with our ability to fall asleep at night. It's important to find the right nap time that works for you and your body's natural rhythms.

While taking a quick nap can be beneficial for your alertness and ability to take on new tasks, it's important to not oversleep. Studies have shown that sleeping longer than 20 minutes can actually have a negative impact on your energy levels and leave you feeling tired for the rest of the day. To avoid this, it's important to set an alarm for a short nap and stick to it. This way, you can reap the benefits of a quick snooze without any negative effects on the rest of your day. So next time you're feeling a little sleepy, set that alarm and enjoy a rejuvenating nap.

As recommended by sleep experts, for those who struggle to fall asleep quickly, there is a simple yet effective trick that can help. It all comes down to controlling your breathing. Begin by finding a comfortable position, closing your eyes, and directing your attention to your breath. Inhale deeply and exhale slowly, setting a gentle and steady rhythm. As you do this, mentally release the tension in all your muscles, starting from your feet and working your way up to the top of your head. This technique can bring about a sense of relaxation and help you drift off to sleep in no time.

Taking a nap can do wonders for our overall productivity and well-being, but it's important to make sure we wake up properly. When your alarm goes off, don't immediately open your eyes. Instead, take a few moments to let your mind slowly wake up. Do some gentle wrist and ankle stretches while mentally preparing for the tasks ahead. Once your body is fully awake, then open your eyes. By following this process, you can start your post-nap period feeling refreshed and ready to tackle the rest of your day.

In order to maintain a healthy and well-rested body, it's important to establish a regular nap schedule. This will create a natural activity/rest cycle that allows for easier sleep and waking patterns. As time goes on, your body will adapt and relax more easily, potentially allowing you to wake up without an alarm and take short, rejuvenating micro-naps of three or four minutes when time is limited. By prioritizing a consistent nap schedule, you can improve your overall energy and productivity levels.

36.   Massage

Massage therapy can be incredibly beneficial in reducing stress, both physically and mentally. Our muscles can hold onto tension and stress after an injury or overuse, leading to increased pain and discomfort. This physical stress can also cause mental stress, as restricted movement and pain can lead to an increase in the hormone cortisol, resulting in feelings of anxiety and depression. While a small amount of stress can be helpful, too much can have negative effects, such as fear of returning to physical activity or self-doubt. Through massage, these physical and mental stresses can be addressed and relieved, promoting overall well-being and a better quality of life.

The massage techniques most commonly used to reduce stress include deep tissue massage, Swedish massage and therapeutic massage.

Deep tissue massage is a highly effective method for reducing stress in the body. This type of massage targets the deeper layers of soft tissues, which are often the source of tension and discomfort. By stretching and spreading the muscle fibres and tissues, a deep tissue massage can relieve built-up tension and promote relaxation. As a result, muscles become more relaxed and mobile, leading to a decrease in pain and stress levels. With its focus on the root causes of stress, a deep tissue massage is an excellent choice for those seeking relief and relaxation.

In today's fast-paced and demanding world, stress has become a common issue for many people. Fortunately, one effective way to reduce stress is through Swedish massage. This type of massage focuses on manipulating the muscles to promote relaxation and ease tension, both physically and mentally. By encouraging the muscles to relax and stretch, Swedish massage can effectively relieve tightness and tension, reducing physical stress. And as we all know, physical stress often leads to mental stress, so by targeting the root cause, Swedish massage can also help to decrease mental stress levels. So, whether you're looking to unwind after a long day or manage chronic stress, Swedish massage can be a valuable tool in your self-care routine.

Therapeutic massage is a popular and effective method for reducing stress and promoting relaxation. By applying gentle pressure to areas of soft tissue, a therapeutic massage aims to alleviate tension and promote a sense of well-being. When relaxation is compromised, stress levels can rise, leading to the build-up of tension, anxiety, and muscular knots. However, a therapeutic massage can help increase local blood flow, which carries positive hormones such as endorphins, serotonin, and dopamine. These hormones have been shown to improve mood and promote relaxation, ultimately reducing stress levels. Furthermore, the increase in blood flow can also help improve tissue elasticity by raising muscle temperature. This increase in elasticity can prevent the formation of muscular knots and further reduce tension, resulting in a decrease in overall stress levels.

Various techniques are used to reduce stress. The techniques most commonly used include:

Deep Strokes

Trigger Pointing

Lymphatic drainage

Deep strokes are a highly effective technique used in massage therapy to reduce stress and tension within the body. This method involves using firm pressure to reach deep within the muscle tissues, targeting both superficial and deeper layers of muscle stress. Often, stress can become trapped within the deeper tissues, causing increased pain and restricted movement. By using deep strokes, the temperature of the muscles is increased, promoting tissue elasticity. This helps to loosen tight muscles and decrease stress and tension. Ultimately, the reduction of stress within the muscles not only leads to a decrease in pain, but also an increase in overall movement and flexibility.

Trigger pointing is a highly effective technique used to reduce stress and relieve pain in the body. It involves targeting specific trigger points, which are located in the centre of muscle fibres, where stress and tension have built up and formed muscular knots. These trigger points can cause referred pain, headaches, and increase mental stress. To perform trigger pointing, the fingers and thumbs are used to apply firm pressure to the trigger point. This pressure triggers an ischemic reaction, restricting blood flow to the area, which then increases when the pressure is released. As the pressure is applied, the trigger point starts to soften, creating a numbing sensation. Once this numbing sensation occurs, more pressure can be applied to the trigger point, depending on its depth and size, or the pressure can be released. By softening and numbing the trigger point, pain and headaches can be reduced, and both mental and physical stress can be relieved. Overall, trigger pointing is a highly beneficial technique for promoting relaxation and reducing stress in the body.

Lymphatic drainage has been proven to be an effective method for reducing stress. By stimulating the lymphatic system, this technique helps remove metabolic wastes more efficiently from the body. These wastes can build up after an injury, surgery, or overuse of a muscle, causing swelling, fatigue, and weakness. These symptoms can not only hinder movement but also prevent injuries from healing properly, leading to frustration and increased mental stress. By receiving a massage that specifically targets the lymphatic system, long and deep strokes are used to flush out these wastes and replace them with healthy oxygen and nutrients. This not only reduces swelling, pain, and restriction but also helps to decrease mental stress, allowing individuals to return to their daily activities with a more relaxed state of mind.

Reducing stress through massage can help in a variety of situations. The situations most commonly helped through reduced stress include:

Acute Pain

Post Injury

Relaxation

When it comes to pain, reducing stress can make a significant difference. Both physical and mental stress can contribute to an increase in pain levels. Physical stress can limit movement and create tension in the body. On the other hand, mental stress can exacerbate existing pain by releasing a hormone called cortisol. This further intensifies pain, creating a cycle of increasing pain and stress. Massage therapy targets both muscle relaxation and mental relaxation to alleviate pain. By increasing temperature and improving muscle flexibility and range of movement, massages promote muscle relaxation. Additionally, they work to flush out cortisol from the body, reducing stress levels and ultimately decreasing pain.

Massage therapy has been shown to have positive effects on reducing stress levels in individuals recovering from an injury. After an injury, various conditions such as swelling, muscle fatigue, and weakness can arise, causing added stress to the individual. This stress can be further exacerbated by the inability to return to exercise or sports and the presence of pain. However, receiving a massage can help to promote relaxation both physically and psychologically. The physical touch of a massage stimulates the release of positive hormones such as endorphins, serotonin, and dopamine, which can lead to a sense of well-being and a positive frame of mind. This not only helps to reduce stress levels but also aids in healing and recovery. By reducing stress and promoting healing, massage therapy can assist individuals in returning to their sports and activities more quickly, ultimately reducing stress even further.

In today's fast-paced world, stress has become a common part of daily life. However, it's important to find ways to reduce stress levels in order to promote relaxation. When stress is high, both physically and mentally, it can prevent the body from reaching a state of relaxation. Tense muscles can contribute to this, as they stay in a contracted state and can cause pain and frustration. This is where massage therapy comes in, as it aims to relieve muscle tension. Through friction between the skin and fingers, massage can increase blood flow to the muscles. This, in turn, raises muscle temperature and increases tissue elasticity, allowing the muscles to relax. And as the body relaxes, mental relaxation also increases, thanks to the decrease in pain and increase in movement. So if you're feeling stressed and in need of some relaxation, consider incorporating massage therapy into your self-care routine.

The physiological effects that most commonly occur during a massage to help reduce stress include increased endorphins, serotonin and dopamine, decreased cortisol and increased tissue elasticity.

Did you know that a massage can do more than just relax your muscles? It can actually have a positive impact on your mental well-being as well. By stimulating the autonomic system, a massage encourages the release of endorphins, serotonin, and dopamine – all of which are neurotransmitters responsible for promoting positive emotions. Endorphins can help relieve anxiety, while serotonin prevents depression and gives a sense of well-being. Dopamine, on the other hand, can increase motivation and prevent self-doubt. When our bodies lack these positive hormones, we may experience stress, anxiety, and feelings of loneliness. That's why a massage is not only physically beneficial but can also improve our overall mood by increasing the levels of these hormones in our bodies.

One of the main benefits of getting a massage is the reduction of stress levels through a decrease in cortisol, a negative hormone released from the adrenal gland when the hypothalamus is stimulated. The adrenal gland, located on top of the kidneys, and the hypothalamus, a part of the brain, work together to release cortisol into the bloodstream, causing an increase in stress, anxiety, and depression. However, cortisol is also responsible for the fight or flight response. Too much cortisol can have negative effects on the body, including increased stress and suppressed immune system. A massage targets and removes excess cortisol from the bloodstream, replacing it with positive hormones such as endorphins, serotonin, and dopamine. By replacing cortisol with these positive hormones, stress levels decrease and the body enters a state of relaxation.

In today's fast-paced and demanding world, stress has become a common issue that affects both our physical and mental well-being. Thankfully, massage therapy has been proven to be an effective method in reducing stress. With a variety of massage types such as deep tissue, Swedish, and therapeutic massage, therapists can use techniques like deep strokes, trigger pointing, and lymphatic drainage to target specific areas and help release tension and promote relaxation. This can be especially helpful in situations such as acute pain, post-injury recovery, and overall relaxation. The physiological effects of massage, such as increased endorphins, serotonin, and dopamine, as well as decreased cortisol levels, all contribute to reducing stress and promoting a sense of calm and well-being.

37. Dark chocolate

Great news for all chocolate enthusiasts! Recent research has revealed that dark chocolate has the ability to alleviate stress and promote good health. In fact, a study has shown that consuming dark chocolate can have a positive impact on stress levels. This promising finding adds to the growing body of evidence that dark chocolate has numerous benefits beyond its delicious taste. With its stress-relieving properties and health benefits, there's no better reason to indulge in some dark chocolate today!

A recent clinical trial published in ACS' Journal of Proteome Research revealed that consuming approximately 40g of dark chocolate per day for two weeks can significantly reduce levels of stress hormones in individuals who report feeling highly stressed. Additionally, the study found that dark chocolate had a positive impact on other biochemical imbalances related to stress. These findings highlight the potential benefits of incorporating dark chocolate into one's diet as a means of managing stress levels and promoting overall well-being. As further research is conducted, dark chocolate may become a recommended dietary addition for those struggling with high levels of stress.

A recent study conducted by Francois-Pierre Martin, Sunil Kochhar, and their colleagues revealed promising results for those struggling with high levels of stress. By examining the effects of daily dark chocolate consumption on volunteers who rated themselves as highly stressed, the study found reductions in stress hormones like cortisol, as well as other stress-related biochemical changes. The study concluded that a daily consumption of 40 grams of dark chocolate for two weeks was enough to positively impact the metabolism of healthy human volunteers. These findings offer a potential solution for individuals seeking natural and delicious ways to manage their stress levels.

As part of the study, the researchers cite growing scientific evidence of more benefits associated with dark chocolate:

Antioxidants and other beneficial substances in dark chocolate may reduce risk factors for heart disease

Dark chocolate's antioxidants may reduce risk factors for other diseases and physical conditions as well
Studies show that dark chocolate may ease emotional stress

This, however, is the first study of its kind that shows, in humans, exactly how dark chocolate may help with stress.

Many of us turn to sweets as a way to cope with stress, but this often leads to weight gain and negative impacts on our health. However, there is some good news for chocolate lovers – dark chocolate has been found to have various health benefits. This is particularly reassuring as the body's stress response can trigger cravings for sweets. By enjoying a small amount of dark chocolate mindfully, it can serve as an effective and enjoyable way to relieve stress without negatively affecting our health. As long as there are no medical reasons preventing individuals from consuming dark chocolate, it can be a beneficial addition to one's diet.

38. Get Out In Nature

Numerous studies have shown that spending time in nature can have a positive impact on our mental and emotional well-being. Whether it's referred to as forest bathing, ecotherapy, mindfulness in nature, green time, or the wilderness cure, there is a growing recognition that humans evolved in the great outdoors and that our brains benefit from reconnecting with nature. Not only can it help to relieve stress and anxiety, but it can also improve our mood and boost feelings of happiness and well-being. So the next time you're feeling overwhelmed or down, consider taking a journey back to nature for some much-needed rejuvenation.

Have you been feeling down lately? A little sluggish, stressed out, or maybe wondering, "What's life all about?"

Here's another question: How much time have you spent in nature lately?

The answer to these two questions might be more closely related than you'd think.

In today's fast-paced world, our lives have become increasingly reliant on technology and the modern conveniences it provides. However, despite these advancements, our brains have largely remained the same as they were when we lived in the savanna. This means that our deep connection with nature still exists and it is essential for our overall well-being. Research has shown that neglecting this connection can have negative effects on our physical and mental health. Therefore, it is important to make time to reconnect with nature and reap the benefits it offers. Taking a break from technology and immersing oneself in the great outdoors can be a powerful way to rejuvenate and recharge the mind and body. So, if possible, make it a priority to spend time in nature and nurture that vital connection for a healthier and happier life.

Depressed? Research has shown that spending time in green, natural spaces can have a positive impact on our mental health. So if you're feeling down, try taking a stroll in the woods or simply enjoying the view of a forest from your hospital room. It's been proven that spending time in nature can combat depression and boost our overall mood. Next time you're feeling blue, consider heading for the hills and soaking up the healing powers of nature. Your mind and body will thank you.

Stressed? Nature has a unique way of captivating our attention without overwhelming us. Instead of abrupt and chaotic scenes, it gently draws us in with its beauty and serenity. The calming effects of nature can soothe our nerves and provide a much-needed respite from the hustle and bustle of everyday life. Its gentle presence invites us to slow down and appreciate the world around us, rather than frazzling our senses with loud and abrupt stimuli. In a world filled with constant noise and distractions, nature offers a peaceful and tranquil escape that can help us find balance and inner peace. Take a moment to immerse yourself in the gentle scenes of nature and experience its calming and restorative powers.

Anxious? It's no secret that exercise has numerous mental benefits, such as reducing anxiety and improving overall well-being. However, recent studies have shown that working out in nature can have even more significant positive effects on mental health compared to indoor exercise. By hitting the trails and surrounding yourself with the beauty of nature, you can experience a heightened sense of relaxation and a decrease in anxiety. So instead of hitting the gym, consider taking your workout outside to reap the best mental benefits.

Self-Involved? When faced with constant worries and negative thoughts, it can be hard to find a way to stop the cycle. However, research has shown that a simple 90-minute walk in nature can significantly reduce activity in the brain that is associated with negative rumination. Instead of dwelling on your problems, take a stroll through a meadow and allow the calming effects of nature to put the brakes on your thoughts. It may be just the break your mind needs to reset and find a more positive perspective. So the next time you find yourself stuck in a cycle of negative thinking, take a step outside and let the beauty of nature do its work.

Fatigued? In today's fast-paced world, multitasking has become a necessary skill in both our personal and professional lives. However, constantly switching between tasks can take a toll on our mental abilities. This is because our prefrontal cortex, the part of our brain responsible for executive functions like memory and decision-making, can only handle so much distraction before it needs a break. This is where spending time in nature can be beneficial. Studies have shown that time spent in nature can restore our mental abilities, such as short-term memory and spatial reasoning, giving our brains the much-needed recharge it needs to tackle the daily demands of multitasking. So next time you feel overwhelmed by a barrage of tasks, consider taking a break in nature to give your brain a boost.

Uninspired? It's no secret that sometimes we need a change of scenery to spark our creativity and problem-solving abilities. And what better place to do that than in nature? Research has shown that spending just four days surrounded by nature can improve problem-solving skills by up to 50%. So, if you're feeling stuck on a big project at work or facing an obstacle in your personal life, why not try taking a break and immersing yourself in the great outdoors? Disconnecting from screens and technology and reconnecting with nature can do wonders for our minds and productivity. So next time you're feeling stuck, try taking a walk in the park or planning a weekend camping trip. You might be surprised at the solutions and inspiration you find in the beauty of nature.

Antisocial? Aside from the obvious benefits of being in nature for our physical and mental health, spending time in nature can also have positive effects on our personal relationships. Research has shown that exposure to natural beauty can lead to more prosocial behaviours, such as increased generosity and empathy. This can be beneficial in fostering stronger and more meaningful connections with those around us. So next time you're feeling stressed or disconnected, try spending some time in nature to not only benefit yourself, but also those in your life.

Disconnected? In today's fast-paced and technology-driven world, it's easy to feel disconnected from our surroundings and the natural world. However, research has shown that spending time in nature can have a significant impact on our mental health and sense of belonging. As humans, we have an innate need to feel like we belong and are part of a larger tribe, and this extends beyond just human relationships. Spending time in nature can provide us with a sense of belonging to the wider world, which is crucial for our mental well-being. Whether it's taking a hike, sitting in a park, or simply admiring the beauty of a tree, reconnecting with nature can help us feel more connected and grounded in the world around us.

Angsty? Life can be overwhelming and confusing at times, leaving us feeling lost and questioning our purpose. However, in moments like these, a dose of awe can serve as a powerful reminder of the wondrous world we live in. Just look to nature, where you can find trees that have been standing for centuries, towering mountains that seem to touch the clouds, and a vast sky filled with countless stars. It's in these moments that we realize just how small we are in comparison to the grandeur of the universe. Nature has a way of leaving us in awe, reminding us of the power and beauty that surrounds us every day. And what could be more powerful than that? So when life gets overwhelming, take a step outside and let the wonder of nature rekindle your sense of purpose and perspective.

39. Good nutrition

Is it true that certain foods worsen anxiety and others have a calming effect?

Living with anxiety can be challenging, as the symptoms can often make you feel unwell. Coping with anxiety may require making significant lifestyle changes, and while there is no diet that can cure anxiety, being mindful of what you eat may offer some relief. It's important to remember that every person's experience with anxiety is unique, so it's essential to find the right combination of strategies that work for you. Some lifestyle changes that may help with managing anxiety include regular exercise, practicing relaxation techniques, and seeking support from loved ones or a therapist. In addition, incorporating a balanced and healthy diet can also play a role in reducing anxiety symptoms. By focusing on a nutrient-dense diet and avoiding foods that may exacerbate anxiety, individuals may find some relief from their symptoms. As always, it's essential to consult with a healthcare professional before making any significant changes to your diet or lifestyle.

Try these steps:

Eat a breakfast that includes some protein. Protein is an essential nutrient that can greatly impact our overall health and well-being. Incorporating protein into our breakfast meals is a simple yet effective way to boost our energy levels and feel fuller longer throughout the day. Not only does protein help stabilize our blood sugar levels, but it also provides our bodies with the necessary building blocks to repair and maintain our muscles, tissues, and organs. This can lead to increased strength, improved immune function, and better overall health. By starting our day with a protein-rich breakfast, we can set ourselves up for success and maintain steady energy levels throughout the day. So next time you reach for that sugary cereal or carb-heavy breakfast option, consider adding some protein to keep you feeling satisfied and energized.

Eat complex carbohydrates. Carbohydrates can increase serotonin levels in the brain, which can have a calming effect. However, it's important to focus on consuming complex carbohydrates, like whole grains, for maximum benefits. This includes foods like oatmeal, quinoa, whole-grain breads, and cereals. It's best to avoid foods high in simple carbohydrates, such as sugary treats and drinks, as these can cause blood sugar spikes and crashes, leading to mood swings and irritability. Remember, balance is key when it comes to incorporating carbohydrates into your diet for optimal mood and overall health.

Drink plenty of water. Proper hydration is crucial for our physical health, but did you know it can also have a significant impact on our mood? Even mild dehydration, which can occur when we are not consuming enough fluids, can lead to irritability, fatigue, and decreased focus. Our brains are made up of mostly water, and when we are dehydrated, it can affect the production of neurotransmitters that regulate our mood. That's why it's essential to stay hydrated throughout the day, not just when we feel thirsty. By keeping a water bottle with you and sipping on it regularly, you can ensure your body and mind stay properly hydrated and in a positive mood.

Limit or avoid alcohol. While alcohol may initially provide a sense of calmness, its effects on the body can quickly turn to restlessness and irritability. As alcohol is processed by the body, it can lead to increased agitation and interfere with the quality of sleep. These negative effects can have a significant impact on daily functioning and overall well-being. It's important to be mindful of alcohol consumption and its potential effects on mood and sleep patterns.

Limit or avoid caffeine. It's no secret that caffeine is a widely used stimulant, but it's important to be mindful of how much you consume and when. While it may provide a temporary boost of energy, it can also lead to feelings of jitteriness and nervousness. Furthermore, caffeine can have a negative impact on your sleep, making it harder to fall asleep and stay asleep. For these reasons, it's important to limit or avoid caffeinated beverages, especially in the afternoon and evening. Instead, opt for non-caffeinated options or stick to a moderate intake of caffeine earlier in the day to avoid potential negative effects on your well-being.

Pay attention to food sensitivities. For some individuals, consuming certain foods or food additives can result in unpleasant physical reactions. These reactions can then trigger shifts in mood, leading to symptoms such as irritability or anxiety. It's important to pay attention to these reactions and make note of any potential triggers, as avoiding these foods can greatly improve one's overall well-being. Additionally, consulting with a healthcare professional can help identify any underlying allergies or sensitivities and develop a personalized plan for managing these symptoms. With the right approach, it is possible to find relief and improve both physical and mental health.

Try to eat healthy, balanced meals. Eating a balanced and nutritious diet is crucial for maintaining both our physical and mental well-being. A key component of this is incorporating plenty of fresh fruits and vegetables into our meals, as well as avoiding overeating. Additionally, including fish high in omega-3 fatty acids, like salmon, in our regular diet can have numerous health benefits. By making these small but impactful changes to our eating habits, we can greatly improve our overall health and well-being.

While changes to your diet and lifestyle can have an impact on your overall mood and well-being, they should not be seen as a substitute for professional treatment for anxiety. It's important to work with a healthcare provider to find the right treatment plan for you. That being said, making small lifestyle changes such as improving sleep habits, increasing social support, practicing stress-reduction techniques, and getting regular exercise can also help alleviate anxiety symptoms. It's important to be patient and give these changes time to take effect, as they may not provide immediate relief. Remember to always consult with a healthcare professional for the best course of action in managing anxiety.

If your anxiety is severe or interferes with your day-to-day activities or enjoyment of life, you may need counselling (psychotherapy), medication or other treatment.

40. Nutritional supplements

Anxiety is a common and often debilitating condition that affects many people. In an effort to find relief, some individuals turn to dietary supplements, believing they may help reduce their symptoms. While there is some evidence to suggest that certain supplements, such as omega-3 fatty acids and magnesium, may have a positive impact on anxiety, it's crucial to understand the facts before incorporating them into your treatment plan. It's important to consult with a healthcare professional before starting any new supplements, as they may interact with other medications and could potentially cause harmful side effects. Furthermore, it's essential to carefully research the supplement and choose a reputable brand, as the supplement industry is not heavily regulated. Understanding the potential benefits and risks of dietary supplements for anxiety is crucial for making informed decisions about your mental health treatment.

L-theanine, an amino acid naturally found in green tea leaves, has been shown to have potential benefits for easing stress and anxiety. In fact, a 2019 review of 9 studies found that taking 200 to 400 milligrams (mg) of L-theanine supplements each day can significantly reduce stress and anxiety levels in individuals facing stressful situations. Additionally, a small 2019 study found that L-theanine may also help alleviate stress-related symptoms and improve sleep quality. Typically available in 200-mg capsules, it is important to start with the lowest possible dose when trying L-theanine and to consult with a healthcare professional before taking more than 400 mg. Whether used for stress management or to promote better sleep, L-theanine may offer a natural and effective solution for those looking to improve their overall well-being.

Ashwagandha, an Ayurvedic herb that has been used in India for centuries, has gained popularity in the United States as a supplement in recent years, particularly for its potential to reduce stress and anxiety. While research into its benefits is still relatively new, a small 2019 study found it to be safe and effective for these purposes. However, due to the limited knowledge on the appropriate dosage, it is best to consult with a healthcare professional before incorporating ashwagandha into your diet. As with any supplement, it is important to be cautious and seek professional guidance for optimal results.

Magnesium is a crucial mineral for overall health, as it is involved in numerous bodily functions such as muscle function, blood pressure regulation, and stress response. This essential mineral also supports metabolism and aids in the utilization of carbohydrates, fats, and amino acids. It is generally safe to take as a supplement, and recent research suggests that it may also benefit those who struggle with anxiety. However, the recommended dosage may vary depending on age and sex, with adult men advised to consume 400 to 420 mg of total magnesium daily, while adult women should aim for 310 to 320 mg a day. It's important to consult with a healthcare professional before starting any new supplement regimen.

Curcumin, a polyphenol compound found in turmeric, has been found to have powerful antioxidant and anti-inflammatory properties. Not only that, but a 2017 review of six studies showed that curcumin also has great anti-anxiety effects and can positively impact depression symptoms. This is significant, considering the analysis was small. Additionally, a 2017 study with 123 participants found that curcumin was particularly effective in reducing symptoms for those with major depressive disorder. This compound has also been shown to reduce anxiety symptoms in individuals with diabetes. With these findings, it's clear that curcumin may have potential as a natural remedy for both depression and anxiety.

Saffron is a spice that has gained popularity in the culinary world for its vibrant colour and distinct flavour. However, it also boasts impressive medicinal properties that should not be overlooked. Loaded with antioxidants, saffron supplements have been shown to improve mood and promote relaxation. In fact, a 2018 review of 100 studies found that saffron, among other herbs, was effective in reducing anxiety. More recent clinical trials have also revealed that saffron can be just as effective as antidepressant medications in treating depression, but with fewer side effects. With its proven benefits for both physical and mental well-being, saffron is a valuable addition to any diet or supplement regimen.

Vitamin D is a crucial nutrient that plays a vital role in maintaining a healthy mind and body. Our bodies naturally produce this vitamin when exposed to sunlight, but it can also be obtained through certain foods or supplements. Research has shown a correlation between low levels of vitamin D and depression, as well as other mood disorders such as anxiety. In fact, a recent study found that vitamin D supplementation can help reduce the severity of anxiety symptoms. It's important to note that the appropriate dosage of vitamin D varies for each individual, depending on their current levels. A doctor can perform a simple test to determine the right dosage for you and ensure that you are getting the right amount of this essential nutrient.

Omega-3s are essential fats with impressive anti-inflammatory properties. Unlike other fats, our bodies cannot produce omega-3s on their own and must obtain them from our diet or through supplements. In fact, a 2018 review of 19 clinical trials showed that omega-3s can significantly reduce symptoms of anxiety in individuals who were treated with omega-3 supplements, as compared to a control group. The review also found that higher doses of omega-3s, at least 2,000 mg per day, were most effective in reducing anxiety symptoms. These findings suggest that incorporating omega-3s into our diet or supplement routine may have significant benefits for our mental health.

Vitamin C is a powerful nutrient that acts as an antioxidant in the body. Not only does it support overall health, but multiple studies have also shown its effectiveness in treating symptoms of anxiety in people of all ages. A 2015 study focused on high school students found that a daily dose of 500 mg of vitamin C for 2 weeks helped reduce anxiety levels. Furthermore, research from 2013 and 2017 has also indicated that vitamin C supplements can provide anxiety relief in people with diabetes and women, respectively. The recommended daily intake of vitamin C varies depending on age, but it can typically be obtained through a balanced diet rich in fruits.

Including vitamin C in your daily routine can be a beneficial addition to support both physical and mental well-being.

Chamomile is a versatile herb that has been used for centuries for its soothing and calming properties. While it is most commonly consumed as a tea, it has also been found to have anti-anxiety and antidepressant effects with regular use. A 2016 study even suggests that chamomile may be beneficial in reducing symptoms of generalized anxiety disorder. However, more research is needed to determine the most effective dosages and forms of chamomile. With its availability in various forms such as capsules, oils, and tea, it's important to carefully follow the directions on the product and consult a healthcare professional for any concerns or questions. Overall, chamomile is a natural option for those seeking relief from anxiety and stress, but it's important to use it safely and responsibly.

41. CBD oil

As numerous studies have demonstrated, CBD oil has proven to be a highly effective treatment for anxiety, depression, and stress. This natural remedy has been shown to offer a multitude of benefits for those struggling with these mental health conditions. Not only does CBD oil provide relief from symptoms, but it also offers a more natural alternative to traditional medications, which can often come with unwanted side effects. Additionally, CBD oil has been found to have a positive impact on other aspects of overall wellness, such as improving sleep and reducing inflammation. With its numerous proven benefits, it's no wonder that CBD oil is becoming increasingly popular as a natural treatment for anxiety, depression, and stress.

In recent years, CBD oil has become increasingly popular due to its effectiveness in alleviating symptoms of anxiety, depression, and stress. As a result, numerous reputable CBD manufacturers have entered the expanding market, all with the well-being of health-conscious consumers in mind. These manufacturers have dedicated themselves to producing high-quality, safe, and effective CBD products, ensuring that consumers can reap the potential benefits of this natural remedy without any risks or concerns. As the demand for CBD continues to grow, it is important for consumers to choose trusted and reliable brands that prioritize their health and wellness.

In the world of CBD, not all manufacturers are created equal. While there are certainly many reputable companies producing high-quality products, there are also numerous sub-par companies looking to make a quick profit by selling ineffective or impure products. This can be disheartening for consumers looking to experience the benefits of CBD, but it's important to remember that not all hope is lost. When searching for quality CBD products, it's crucial to do thorough research and carefully consider the manufacturer. By keeping this in mind, you can ensure that you are investing in safe and effective products from a reputable company. Don't let the abundance of lower-quality options deter you from experiencing the potential benefits of CBD.

CBD, or cannabidiol, has been shown to have positive effects on anxiety, depression, and stress by interacting with over 65 areas within the body. As a professional, it's important to understand how CBD works and its potential benefits for clients experiencing these mental health concerns. By targeting specific areas within the body, CBD can help regulate and balance mood, reduce symptoms of anxiety and depression, and promote a sense of calm and relaxation. This natural and non-psychoactive compound is becoming increasingly popular as a treatment option for mental health, and it's important for professionals to stay informed on its uses and potential benefits.

Recent research studies have found that CBD, or cannabidiol, has shown promise in reducing anxiety through various mechanisms. One of these is through the stimulation of neural regeneration and neurotransmitter systems, leading to an overall positive effect on mood and stress levels. CBD has also been found to regulate the endocannabinoid system, which can become dysregulated through chronic stress. This suggests that CBD could potentially be an effective natural remedy for anxiety, with minimal side effects compared to traditional medications. As more research is conducted, we hope to gain a deeper understanding of how CBD can be used to help manage anxiety and improve overall mental health.

In addition to its numerous benefits for physical health, CBD has also shown promising results in improving mental health. Specifically, CBD has been found to bind to serotonin receptors, including the 5-HT1A receptor, which is responsible for anxiety disorders. This interaction allows CBD to effectively reduce anxiety and promote feelings of calm and relaxation, often with comparable or even better results than prescription anti-anxiety medications. With its natural and non-addictive properties, CBD offers a potential alternative for those seeking relief from anxiety without the negative side effects of traditional medications.

Looking for the highest quality CBD oil? Look no further than mywaycbd.com. Our products are crafted with care and undergo rigorous testing to ensure the utmost quality and effectiveness. And for a limited time, use the code BLISS for 20% off your purchase.

42. Time management

As professionals, it's crucial to master time management in order to effectively handle a heavy workload without experiencing excessive stress. Good time management skills not only help to alleviate immediate stress, but also reduce long-term stress by providing a sense of direction when faced with a heavy workload. By effectively managing your time, you can prioritize tasks and allocate the necessary time and resources to complete them, reducing the feeling of being overwhelmed. Time management also allows for more efficient use of time, increasing productivity and minimizing stress levels in the long run. Therefore, mastering time management is a key component of maintaining a healthy work-life balance and ensuring success in your professional endeavours.

Being in control of our time is crucial for our productivity and overall satisfaction with work and life. By using our time efficiently, we can make the most of our work hours and have more time to relax and enjoy other aspects of life. It's all about finding a balance and managing our time effectively. This not only benefits us professionally, but also personally. When we are able to accomplish our tasks in a timely and organized manner, we can feel more fulfilled and accomplished, leading to a more positive outlook on work and life. So let's take control of our time and strive for productivity and balance.

In the fast-paced world we live in, it's no surprise that poor time management can lead to a great deal of stress. We've all experienced that overwhelming feeling of having too much to do and not enough time to do it. This can lead to panic, anxiety, and a loss of focus. It's worth noting that even when our to-do lists may seem manageable, we can still feel this sense of unease and pressure. In order to reduce stress levels and maintain productivity, it's crucial to effectively manage our time and prioritize tasks. This will not only help us accomplish more, but also allow us to maintain a sense of calm and control in our daily lives.

Symptoms of stress caused by poor time management:
1.Irritability and mood swings

2. Tiredness and fatigue
3. Inability to focus or concentrate. Do you ever feel like you are just trying to get yourself through the day?
4. Mental block, memory lapses and forgetfulness.
5. Lack of, or loss of, sleep
6. At worst, withdrawal and depression

In a professional setting, managing your time is crucial for productivity and success. Failing to do so can lead to a lack of clarity and direction, causing you to prioritize tasks based on what is immediately in front of you or in response to others' demands. This can result in neglecting important tasks and hindering progress on your own work. It is essential to prioritize and manage your time effectively in order to achieve your goals and maintain a productive workflow. This means setting aside distractions and staying focused on the tasks that truly matter. By doing so, you can avoid falling behind and ensure that your work is completed efficiently and effectively.

As long as you commit to taking action time management is easy. Simple steps can result in more effective management of your time. These can include:
1. Better planning
2. Better prioritising
3. Delegating tasks to others
4. Controlling your environment

43. Setting boundaries

Creating boundaries in relationships can be a challenging process. It requires openly communicating your needs and limits to others, which can be stressful for those who are not used to setting boundaries. This can be especially difficult when trying to change existing boundaries with people who are accustomed to a certain level of interaction. Children and others may also test boundaries, adding to the stress of the situation. Conflict can also contribute to increased stress levels. However, the benefits of setting and enforcing boundaries are significant. It leads to relationships with greater levels of mutual respect, meets the needs of all parties involved, and reduces overall stress for everyone. By setting and maintaining healthy boundaries, we can create more positive and fulfilling relationships in our lives.

When it comes to setting boundaries, it's crucial to have a clear understanding of your own personal boundaries. This involves recognizing your level of comfort with people getting physically close to you or taking certain liberties with you. Often, the first sign that your boundaries have been crossed is a feeling of discomfort. However, it's important to remember that everyone has different boundaries, so what may bother someone else may not bother you and vice versa. To effectively communicate your boundaries to others, it's important to be aware of them yourself. The following guidelines can help you become more conscious of your own personal boundaries.

Signs You Need to Work on Boundaries

You feel resentful of people asking too much of you, and it seems to happen often.

You find yourself saying yes to things you'd rather not do, just to avoid upsetting or disappointing others.

You find yourself feeling resentful because you are doing more for others than they are doing for you.

You tend to keep most people at an arm's length because you are afraid of letting people get too close and overwhelming you.

You find yourself feeling that most of what you do is for other people—and they may not even appreciate it that much.

The stress you feel from disappointing others is greater than the stress of doing things that inconvenience or drain you in an effort to please them.

There are additional questions you should ask yourself when you are looking at specific choices you can make, rather than your feelings in general, that can help you to decide whether or not a boundary needs to be set. The following questions can help you to clarify your boundaries in specific situations, and navigate through future ones:

If nobody would be disappointed, would you prefer to say yes or no?

Looking at all the benefits and costs of this situation (both tangible and intangible), is it worth the effort to say yes?

Would you feel comfortable posing the same request to someone else?

If people would be upset with you if you said no, do you truly feel that they are coming from a respectful, reasonable place? (And, if not, might it be time to start setting some limits?)

Is this a precedent you want to set? (And, if not, where would be a reasonable place to draw the line?)

Think of someone you feel has very healthy boundaries—the kind you would like to emulate. How do you think they would respond in this situation?

Setting boundaries can be a challenging process, and it often involves negotiation and communication with others. Once we become aware of our own personal comfort zones, we can decide if we want to establish boundaries. However, this is not always a straightforward process. People may have different boundaries that may not align, and they may try to push for greater distance or closeness for their own reasons. In some cases, attempting to change boundaries from the current norm may elicit reactions from others, causing them to reinforce existing boundaries in ways that may make us uncomfortable. This is why setting boundaries can often be a struggle, but it is an important step in maintaining healthy relationships.

In order to maintain healthy relationships, it is essential to set boundaries that not only consider our own needs, but also the needs and reactions of others. This requires a level of thoughtfulness and circumspection, as we must balance our own desires with the potential impact on those around us. By setting boundaries, we can communicate our needs effectively and create a sense of mutual respect and understanding in our relationships. This can help to prevent conflicts and promote overall well-being for ourselves and those we interact with. Ultimately, setting boundaries is a crucial aspect of self-care and maintaining healthy relationships.

The questions to ask yourself when discovering where your personal boundaries lie are different from the questions may ask yourself when deciding where to actually set your boundaries in specific situations, because they take into account practical factors like the "cost" of setting boundaries. They also allow you to be clear on issues such as guilt (should you feel guilty?) and motivation (is it worth it?) so you can move forward with the least amount of stress.

Here are some questions to ask yourself:

What is fair here?

If you were in the position of the other person, would your solution still appear to be fair?

Have you committed to this, or is this an expectation that the other person is placing on you?

Is there another solution here that could be more win-win?

Does the act of making a change or setting a boundary create more stress than it might alleviate in the long run?

When you imagine the results a year from now, do you get a sense that this would be a better solution than what you have now?

If you are setting a boundary and you feel the other person is unreasonable in fighting the boundary, and you are willing to let the relationship go rather than feel hurt by the boundary mismatch?

When it comes to setting boundaries, it's natural to prioritize our own feelings and the consequences we will have to live with. After all, it's our own lives that will be impacted by the decisions we make. However, it's important to also consider the feelings of others and how our boundaries may affect them. This requires self-reflection and careful consideration of where we draw the line. Each person has their own comfort levels when it comes to boundaries, but it's helpful to ask ourselves some important questions to guide our decision-making. Once we have established our boundaries, implementing strategies and assertive communication techniques can lead to positive results in our relationships and lives.

44. Build resilience

In today's fast-paced world, resilience is more important than ever. It is the ability to withstand pressure and bounce back from adversity without experiencing negative effects. This skill can be developed by incorporating healthy habits into your lifestyle and by changing your mindset and behaviour in challenging situations. By taking care of your physical, mental, and emotional well-being, you can increase your resilience and better handle stress. This includes practicing self-care, setting boundaries, and seeking support when needed. Additionally, reframing your thoughts and reactions to stressful events can help you build a stronger resilience muscle. With determination and effort, you can become more resilient and better equipped to handle the demands of daily life.

To help build your resilience to pressure and stress, try:

increasing the amount of exercise, you do

eating a healthy, balanced diet

making sure you get plenty of sleep

cutting down on caffeine and alcohol

practising assertiveness and learning when to say no to tasks you can't handle

asking for help when you begin to feel under pressure

Managing your workload and time effectively is crucial for reducing stress in the workplace. It's important to assess your workload each day and break it down into small, achievable goals to avoid feeling overwhelmed. Tackling harder tasks early on can also help prevent procrastination and further stress. It's important to be realistic about the time it will take to complete tasks and to only commit to what you can realistically handle. By following these strategies, you can keep stress at bay and improve your overall productivity and well-being.

In today's fast-paced world, it's essential to have strong resilience and coping skills to manage stress. Luckily, there are many free resources available to help you build these skills, such as mindfulness, relaxation, and time management apps and websites. Take some time to explore and find the right fit for you.

Additionally, our blog offers valuable insights on mindfulness and relaxation that may be beneficial to you. Remember, investing in your well-being is always a worthwhile endeavour.

45. Talking

Stress can often feel overwhelming and it's easy to get caught up in our own thoughts and worries. That's why it's important to have a support system and to talk to someone about our stressors. Whether it's a presentation, a trip, or a big event, having someone to confide in can provide significant relief. This person can offer advice, understanding, and support because they have either experienced the same situation or are going through it with you. So, if you're feeling stressed, don't be afraid to reach out and talk to someone who can offer you comfort and guidance. It can make a world of difference.

The impact of human connection on stress relief is significant, according to a study led by Sarah Townsend, an assistant professor at USC Marshall School of Business. In her research, she found that the most effective form of stress relief comes from genuine interaction with someone who not only understands your emotions and responses, but also shares them in the moment. This connection with another person can provide measurable relief from stress, highlighting the importance of human relationships in our well-being. Whether it's a friend, family member, or colleague, taking the time to connect and empathize with others can have a powerful impact on our stress levels.

Townsend and her team conducted a study where participants were paired up based on their emotional similarity and were asked to give a speech while being recorded. Prior to the presentation, each pair was instructed to discuss their feelings with one another. Throughout this process, the participants' cortisol levels were measured and recorded. The purpose of this study was to understand how the stress hormone, cortisol, is affected by emotional support and discussion before a high-pressure task. This study sheds light on the importance of emotional support and communication in reducing stress levels in high-pressure situations.

The study published in Social Psychological and Personality Science found that engaging in conversation with someone who is emotionally similar can act as a buffer against the high levels of stress that come with preparing for a speech. This discovery highlights the importance of finding a partner who shares similar emotions and can provide a sense of support and calm during potentially stressful situations. This can be particularly beneficial for individuals who struggle with public speaking and may experience heightened levels of anxiety. So, the next time you have to prepare for a speech, consider finding an emotionally similar partner to help ease the stress and carry on with confidence.

Conclusion

According to recent statistics, there has been a significant increase in stress levels among Americans, with 31% reporting a rise in their stress levels in just the past year (The American Psychological Association, 2018). This is a concerning trend that can have serious impacts on individuals' mental and physical well-being. It is crucial that we address this issue and find ways to effectively manage and reduce stress in our daily lives. From implementing self-care practices to seeking professional help, there are many resources available to help combat the effects of stress. By acknowledging the prevalence of stress and taking steps to address it, we can work towards creating a healthier and happier society.

As individuals, it's important to pay attention to the warning signs that indicate high levels of stress, such as headaches, stomach knots, and racing thoughts. These signals are our internal alarm bells, reminding us to take action before our stress becomes unmanageable. The good news is that we have the ability to respond and implement a realistic stress management plan. With the abundance of resources available, it's important to listen to our bodies and adapt a plan that works best for us from the extensive list of strategies available. By taking action and managing our stress, we can improve our overall well-being and lead happier, healthier lives.

Hans Selye put it right when he said:

"It's not stress that kills us; it is our reaction to it."

So How will you manage your stress?

Try out the different tips and techniques we've discussed here and see what works best for you. If you have your own techniques that aren't listed here, please do let me know so I can keep growing the list.

Even though we may know what can help alleviate stress and anxiety, it can be challenging to remember and implement these practices in moments of overwhelming emotions. It's important to take the time to do research and find coping mechanisms that work for you. Whether it's deep breathing exercises, talking to a friend or therapist, or engaging in a favourite hobby, it's crucial to have these tools at hand when stress and anxiety arise. By actively practicing and incorporating these methods into our daily lives, we can better manage our stress and anxiety levels, leading to improved overall well-being.